The
Grosset
Encyclopedia
of
NATURAL MEDICINE

The Grosset Encyclopedia of

NATURAL MEDICINE

Robert Thomson

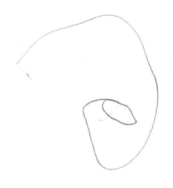

Grosset & Dunlap
A Filmways Company
Publishers   New York

This book is dedicated to
William Morrison Thomson
my brother

Also by Robert Thomson:
Natural Medicine

Published simultaneously in Canada
Library of Congress catalog card number: 79-56186
ISBN 0-448-14897-8
First printing 1980
Printed in the United States of America

Contents

Notice

The intended use of this book among general readers does not include self-treatment of complicated diseases. Simple remedies are frequently used in the initial stages of physiological imbalance, when a person is not in a serious stage of ill health.

It cannot be stressed enough, however, that in the case of serious illness, a physician or other medical adviser should be consulted.

بسم الله الرحمن الرحيم

The Persian calligraphy that opens the Introduction is an in-
vocation written in a stylized form, which is used by all *hakims*
to commence any written work. It reads, *"Bismallah Ir-rahman,
Ir-rahim,"* which means, "In the name of Allah, Most Gracious, Most
Merciful." It was drawn by Enayat Shahrani of Badakshan.
 May God grant you Peace, Health, and Long Life.

Introduction

The story of the researching, compiling, and writing of this Encyclopedia
should be set forth in brief detail, so that those who read the book may have an
idea of how the author and editor hope it may be used.
 For the past ten years, I have been involved in researching and writing on
the subjects of natural therapeutics, herbology, alternative cancer therapies,
nutrition, and related subjects. Included in my work have been research periods in the Near East and India, where I had the opportunity to study, first-
hand, cultures in which treatment by natural means forms the basis of all medical treatment.
 When I returned from Afghanistan in 1976 after a year's stay as a Fulbright
research scholar, I was compelled to begin to organize, in a formal way, all my
library and research holdings on natural medical subjects, as part of the process
of writing a text on classic herbal medicine. As I did so, I became overwhelmed
by the sheer magnitude of books, articles, dissertations, and related published
materials on thousands of different topics. I found myself using a book for
reference only once or twice per year, and constantly having to pore labori-
ously over dozens of books to locate some singular piece of information comprising only a few pages, or even a paragraph, of an individual book.
 At this same time, in the middle 1970s, there began a tremendous increase
of interest in all subjects allied with natural medicine—Chinese acupuncture,
iridology, reflexology, herbology, applied kinesiology—and many other rediscovered or revived therapies. In fact, the proliferation of practitioners and research in these areas has become so great that there exists, at the present time,
a real potential for confusion because of the jumble of vernaculars and termi-
nologies, which sometimes even mislead the general public—who, after all,
usually have little or no formal education in medical subjects of any kind.
 Thus, I sensed a need that had to be filled, and with no particular intention

of writing a full-blown encyclopedia, I began to construct my own files into a general subject listing of all the topics that seemed appropriate. Over the next two years, I eventually arrived at alphabetical files covering more than a thousand topic headings for natural therapeutics.

In 1977 I was contacted by Grosset & Dunlap inquiring if I would be interested in working with them in constructing an encyclopedia of Natural Medicine, as, quite independently of my work, they had been aware of the need for such a volume themselves.

In the next few months, working together, we amassed an exhaustive grouping of six hundred subject listings for inclusion and began to extend our areas of research to select appropriate illustrations and other factual data. Often, the scope of the project seemed to be so large as to test our resolve.

The book which has resulted is, in my judgment, the most comprehensive volume on the subject of natural medicine ever compiled. And, in saying so, I also realize immediately the limitations which will surely occur to anyone reading it.

The philosophy which guided the selection of entries was to present an unbiased review of the origin and essence of the treatment or the substance of each entry, along with any superior and accepted text on the subject. In some cases, we were able also to include information on national organizations which could be contacted for practitioners of a specific therapy or for additional information.

There is no single theory of medicine or health care which we wish to espouse. The entries are intentionally devoid of any personal references or individual testimonies to the effectiveness of a therapy or substance. While this book should not be considered as scholarly or academic in the true sense of those words, it is as unbiased as possible.

It is my hope that medical doctors, naturopaths, chiropractors, naprapaths, homeopaths, all the unorthodox practitioners, educators, and the general public will find a quick, succinct reference to virtually any subject or topic which may occur in the course of extending their knowledge of natural therapeutics.

The Encyclopedia is, in this first edition, a beginning and tentative effort to bring some organization to a disorganized field, and each reader who has comments on the entries or wishes to make suggestions for new entries in future editions is encouraged to submit any information for consideration or inclusion in later editions.

Since this book is one of general information and is intended for use by members of many different healing systems—which are often in "competition" with one another or who reject the theories of one another—there are no mentions or suggestions of specific remedies for diseases (or any other name for unbalanced conditions of the human body). The approach is an attempt to demonstrate to all persons, the patients and the practitioners, that there is much more regarding natural therapies about which to agree than to argue. And, in using and learning from this Encyclopedia, it is hoped that a new spirit of cooperation can be instilled into everyone seeking the same goal—maximizing the health of the general public.

In selecting material for inclusion in this book, and in editing and writing many entries, it is obvious that I have been assisted by a very great number of persons, many of whom are credited in the text. Still, there were many others who assisted—by their direct concern; by sharing, in the form of written correspondence, suggestions as to style and format; and by donating their expertise in specific cases.

In a most profound sense, we are living in one of the most exciting, challenging, and historic times for medicine, in which the advances are most startling and the challenges most severe. Regardless of which system of healing is employed, the one vital fact is that the human body itself is the actual healing mechanism, and that whatever therapy is used, such measures are only employed to assist the body in its own self-healing role. If this point of view is to be accepted, then it is only by each person assuming responsibility for his or her own health that true happiness and freedom from pain and suffering can be achieved. It is with this understanding and in this spirit that this Encyclopedia is offered, with the hope that it may extend the lives and health of those who choose to use the information it presents.

At the same time, it must be remembered that physicians and others trained in the healing arts are skilled not only in identifying the sources of disease, but in guiding one through the often difficult pathway back to health. If you are suffering from illness, such persons should be consulted and their advice considered seriously.

It is sincerely hoped that this book will increase your understanding of the state of your health, and that we shall be able to continue and expand this volume in future years to keep pace with this most remarkable health movement.

> Robert Thomson, N.D., D.N.
> (Hakim G. M. Chishti)
> Tucson, Arizona

The
Grosset
Encyclopedia
of
NATURAL
MEDICINE

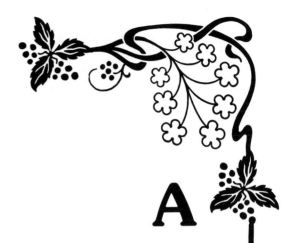

A

Vitamin A

A growth vitamin especially important to children. Lack of vitamin A is felt to be responsible for eye problems, for retardation of growth, and for the diseases *keratemalacia* and *xerophthalmia*. Vitamin A was first isolated in 1913 by a scientist at Yale University, who found it in butterfat. The body cannot store vitamin A, so foods containing this vitamin must be consumed each day, with the average person requiring about 5,000 International Units (IUs) daily. Foods especially rich in vitamin A are raw milk, cod liver oil (30,000 IUs per gram), egg yolk, butter, cream, celery, lettuce, spinach, liver, and heart and kidneys of all animals.

Acacia (Gum Arabic) *Acacia senegal*

The best medicinal gum arabic is a gummy exudate from the *Acacia senegal*. There are few physiological properties; it is most often used as a vehicle and in the manufacture of natural inks.

Acetic Acid

There are two forms: glacial acetic acid and dilute acetic acid. Both are made from a 36 percent solution of acetic acid. Glacial acetic acid is a powerful escharotic. Dilute acetic acid contains about 6 percent acid, about like vinegar. It is sedative and astringent, used for treating superficial skin irritations, night sweats, and epistaxis, and in lotions.

Acetone

A colorless liquid which, in health, may be present in the urine in small quantities. It is formed in the system by decomposition of albuminoid substances. It is found in excessive amounts in the urine and blood in diabetes, autointoxication, starvation, and some fevers. If it is found during pregnancy, it may indicate a dead fetus.

Acid- and Alkali-Producing Foods

As foods are burned up in the body, they leave behind an ash, which is either acidic or alkaline. An increase of acidity is recognized as a principal cause of many disorders. The relative value of acid and alkali is used in choosing foods which decrease the acidity of the body.

The table shows values in selecting foods to combat the tendency toward acidity of the system.

Acid-Producing Foods (representing the total cc. of acidity over base, *per 100 gr.*)		*Alkaline-Producing Foods* (representing the total cc. of alkalinity over base, *per 100 gr.*)	
bread, white	2.7	almonds	12.38
bread, whole wheat	3.0	apples	3.78
corn	5.95	asparagus	.81
crackers	7.81	bananas	5.56
eggs	11.1	beans, dried	23.87
egg white	5.24	beans, lima	41.65
egg yolk	26.69	beets	10.86
fish, haddock	16.07	cabbage	4.34
fish, pike	11.81	carrots	10.82
meat, beef, lean	13.91	cauliflower	5.33
meat, pork, lean	11.87	celery	7.78
meat, chicken	17.01	chestnuts	7.42
meat, veal	13.52	currants	5.97
oysters	30.0	lemons	7.37
oatmeal	12.93	lettuce	7.37
peanuts	3.9	milk, cow's	2.37
rice	8.1	muskmelon	7.47
The ash of some of these foods is alkaline in nature, but because they contain hippuric acid, they increase the acidity of the body.		oranges	5.61
		peaches	5.04
		pears, dried	7.07
		potatoes	7.19
		radishes	2.87
		raisins	23.67
		turnips	2.68

Aconite *(Aconitum Napellus)*

The tuberous root of *Aconitum napellus,* aconite root is alternately called Monk's hood, Wolf's bane, and Blue rocket. It is bitter and pungent in taste, and causes numbness and tingling when applied to the mouth or lips.

Medicinal aconite is used as a circulatory, respiratory, and cardiac depressant. It is antipyretic, diaphoretic, and diuretic. Often used in the initial stages of inflammation; highly beneficial in fevers, acute throat infections, and inflammations of the respiratory organs.

Acupressure

A derivative of the Chinese science of acupuncture, utilizing compression of blood vessels and tissues to adjust energy, whereby relief of symptoms occurs. The term *meridian therapy* is used to denote the application of stimulation to acupuncture meridians in the field of applied kinesiology. George Goodheart, D.C., developed the science of applied kinesiology, synthesizing the use of chiropractic knowledge with acupressure techniques applied by digital stimulation. (See also *Applied Kinesiology.*)

Acupuncture

The puncture of the skin or tissues by one or more needles for relief of pain was recorded as many as five thousand years ago in China, in *The Yellow Emperor's Classic of Internal Medicine.* Acupuncture became famous in the West in the 1950s, after Chinese doctors introduced it in hospitals and private practice.

The medical philosophy underlying acupuncture is that of *Tch'i,* or "life energy," which may be positive, called Yang, or negative, called Yin. The interplay of these two elements is carried on through the main organs and along pathways under the skin called meridians. In disease, there is an interruption or blockage of this flow. The aim of acupuncture is to restore the free flow of this energy by inserting needles into the affected meridian. The affected center is determined by means of a diagnosis of the pulse (see pulse diagnosis). Acupuncture became popular in France at the turn of the twentieth century, and it is accepted in practice even in orthodox hospitals in all of Europe and the United States. The chart shows the acupuncture points for the head and front of the body.

The procedure of acupuncture is to use needles of pure gold, copper, or silver and insert them lightly at the specific points where a blockage of the flow of *Tch'i* is determined to exist. With a competent therapist, there is no discom-

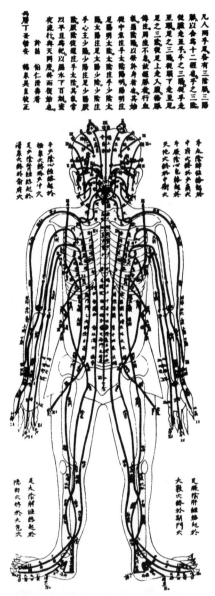

In the Chinese system of acupuncture, the pathways of energy flow (called meridians) *are charted for the entire body.*

fort at all. The needles set up a current along the line of the meridian, which is transmitted to the central nervous system, causing an effect in a corresponding part of the body. The patient is conscious and usually allowed to watch the procedure.

Adrenalin (Epinephrine)

The chief active secretion by the medulla of the adrenal gland, and the most powerful astringent and blood regulator known. In the past, it was used in conjunction with cocaine to increase the effect of anesthesia.

Adrenalin injected into the bloodstream causes a constriction of the blood vessels and an increase in blood pressure; adrenalin is known to have a function in the thermal regulation of the body.

Air (Inspired and Expired)

The composition of the air drawn into the lungs to sustain life (atmospheric air) and the air which is expired after processing by the body is compared in the table below:

	Inspired Air	*Expired Air*
oxygen	20.96 vols.%	16.6 vols.%
nitrogen	70.9 vols.%	79.0 vols.%
carbon dioxide	0.04 vols.%	4.4 vols.%
water vapor	variable	saturated
other gases	rare	$H.NH_4CH_4$
volume	varies	diminished
bacteria	always	none
dust	always	none

Albumin

Albumins are simple proteins soluble in water and coagulated by heat. Albumin present in the urine in any great quantity often means damage or degeneration of the kidneys. However, a temporary albuminuria may appear during adolescence or following extreme exercise, nervous stimulation, or cold. Examples of albumins are those in egg white, lactalbumin in milk, and serum albumin in blood.

Alexander Method

The Alexander Method is based on the principle that conditions of stress often evident in modern life deprive persons, from childhood on, of the natural use of their bodies, thus resulting in many health problems of posture and nervous and tension diseases.

Born in Tasmania in 1869 (d. 1955 in London), Frederick Matthias Alexander developed his theory to restore the use of his voice, which he lost while working as an actor. He observed himself in a mirror and noted that he could consciously control and "restrain" certain facial muscles. He related this principle to other areas of the body as well. His theory and teachings were presented in the 1930s in his book, *The Use of the Self* (New York: Dutton, 1932), which attracted many prominent persons to his mode of health care. The Alexander Method of training the body by conscious application is in use in England up to the present time.

Alfalfa *(Medicago sativa)*

A perennial herbaceous plant native to Asia and imported and domesticated in the United States in the mid-1850s; alfalfa was discovered and named the Father of all Foods by the Arabs, probably due to the presence of so many vital nutrients such as calcium, magnesium, phosphorus, potassium, and all the known vitamins. It has been applied with success both internally and externally to all parts of the body for maintaining and restoring health.

Alkalies (Alkali Reserve)

Alkalies are elements of the group having one valence electron. Potash and soda are examples of alkalies, which can cause severe caustic symptoms if taken in undiluted form. Alkalies operate in the human body to help maintain the stability of the pH in the blood when a strong acid is introduced. The principal buffers which maintain this balance are sodium bicarbonate, disodium phosphate, and the plasma proteins.

The antidote for alkali poisoning is to administer dilute acids, such as citrus, or vinegar and water.

Alkaloids

These are all nitrogenous vegetable compounds of basic and alkaline character, or their derivatives from which bases can be isolated. They are the chief constituents of the active principle of poisons or vegetable drugs employed as medicines. The best known alkaloid, perhaps, is cocaine, an alkaloid of the coca plant. Alkaloids containing no oxygen are generally liquid and volatile. Nicotine is another example.

Almond *(Amygdala amara)*

There are two varieties of *Amygdala amara* ("bitter almond"). A poisonous substance, hydrocyanic acid, is obtained by fermenting the bitter, but not the sweet, almond.

The oil and the saccharin constituents of almonds can be made into bread for diabetics. The emulsion of the oil is used as a vehicle in cough mixtures. It is sedative to the skin, and has been used in treating a variety of diseases, such as gonorrhea.

The most dramatic application of *Amygdala* in recent years has been in the treatment of cancer in all its forms. Synthesized as nitriloside (see *Laetrile*), it has been shown to reduce or eliminate pain in terminal cancer patients, effect an improvement in sense of well-being, and, in some cases, promote a total remission of tumors. The synthetic form has been legalized in several states, and scientific experimentation is under way to verify the results obtained. The ash of apricot kernels, which also contains amygdalin, has long been used in tumors of the skin, and is a regular part of the diet among the Hunzas and other people who have little or no incidence of cancer.

Aloe *(Aloe vera)*

Aloe is a genus with two hundred species comprised mainly of South African succulents. It has been used in healing for two thousand years, and thrives in warm areas of the United States, from Florida to southwest Arizona and California. It is *not* recommended in cases of degeneration of the liver or gall bladder, during pregnancy or menstruation, or for piles.

The inspissated juice of several varieties of the *Aloe vera* plant are used in treatment of burns. Its properties are said to be due to the presence of *aloin,* a bitter principle and tonic astringent used in treatment of amenorrhea, chronic constipation, and atonic dyspepsia. It is also an emmenagogue, an anthelmintic and a cholagogue.

Alteratives

Certain remedies that alter the course of morbid conditions in some way not fully understood by science, but perhaps by promoting metabolism. The principal alteratives, although there are many, include: antimony, sulphur, sanguinaria, iodine, stillingia, sarsaparilla, cod liver oil, red clover, burdock root, chaparral, and garlic. They are used in a wide range of conditions, often in combination with a stimulant herb, such as cayenne, to sustain the effect.

Anise *(Pimpinella anisum)*

The fruit of *Pimpinella anisum* is slightly stimulant to the heart. Because it liquefies bronchial secretions, it is frequently employed in cough mixtures. In ancient times, anise was used in the East as payment for taxes, and it has been in use in Europe for many centuries as a flavoring in cakes and desserts. Its active principle is the volatile oil *anethol*. The majority of anise oil employed in pharmacy is derived from the star anise of China. It is carminative and pectoral, and in addition to its use in cough treatment, it is used for colic and flatulence in infants, and to increase milk flow in nursing mothers. Oil of anise also repels insects, especially when mixed with oil of sassafras and carbolic oil.

Anthelmintics

Agents that destroy (vermicides) or cause the expulsion (vermifuges) of intestinal worms. Among the herbs used to prevent or destroy worms in the excretory passages are: elecampane, goldenrod, horseradish, hydrangea, lily-of-the-valley, pepo, senna, uva-ursi, wild violet, and wormwood.

Herbs which prevent the excessive secretion of intestinal mucus—the medium for worms—are known as the bitter tonic herbs.

Antimony

A nonmetal having a metallic lustre, antimony is rarely used in Western medicine. It is marketed as a cosmetic in the United States under the name kohl, and in Muslim cultures of the East is used by women as a decorative application to the eyes. Often applied to the eyes of infants, it has a slightly antiseptic quality.

Antiperiodics

Remedies that prevent or greatly lessen the severity of the seizures associated with certain periodic febrile (fever) diseases. Possibly they work by arresting the development of successive crops of pathogenic organisms. The principal ones are: eucalyptus, cinchona bark, iodine, skullcap, Peruvian bark, rue, senna, red raspbelly, and dodder.

Antiphlogistics

Measures and remedies that are regarded as having some specific action in reducing or preventing the progress of the inflammatory process. The chief antiphlogistics are: arnica, balm of Gilead, blue cohosh, hops, ice, burdock root, chamomile, cayenne, chaparral, sandalwood, garlic, white pond lily, lobelia, slippery elm bark, and wormwood.

Measures include rest, venesection, local depletion, purgation, counterirritation, and cold packs.

Antiphlogistics are nearly all *contraindicated* in the presence of tissues whose vitality is impaired through previous disease conditions.

Antipyretics

Agents that reduce high body temperature. This may be done by several different actions working in two principal ways: (1) lessening production of heat by slowing tissue change or reducing circulation, and (2) promoting loss of heat by dilating the cutaneous vessels and increasing exposure to sunlight; producing perspiration and its evaporation, or abstracting heat from the body.

The chief antipyretics are cold baths, aconite, cold drinks, wet packs, camphor, quinine, eucalyptol, and wild indigo.

Antiseptics

Agents that arrest the development of the microorganisms that produce decomposition. Herbs are often made into solutions for this purpose. A *disinfectant* is a solution that is stronger than that required for antiseptic action; thus it is *germicidal*. All disinfectants are germicidal. The principal antiseptics are:

anise oil	echinacea	olive leaves
cassia	eucalyptus	peppermint
cayenne	garlic	quince seeds
clove oil	golden seal	sandalwood
coffee	lily-of-the-valley	tobacco
comfrey	mullein	witch hazel
condurango root	myrrh	wormwood

Apiarist

One who manages one or more yards of bees (apiary).

Apis mellifera (Latin)

Honey bee.

Apple Cider Vinegar

Dr. D. C. Jarvis, in his book *Folk Medicine* (New York: Holt, Rinehart and Winston, 1958; Fawcett World, 1969), notes that inhabitants of Vermont often consume apple cider vinegar as a remedy for many conditions of the body. He recommends its use—especially for relief of arthritis—because it contains a large amount of the mineral salt potassium. Jarvis's dosage is one teaspoon to a glass of water, until one is accustomed to the taste. It was the custom in the 1920s for allopathic physicians to give doses of dilute acetic acid (vinegar) to anemic patients. Adding honey to the liquid is said to improve its beneficial effects.

Apple cider vinegar preferable to distilled spirits as a preservative, is also used as a base in the preparation of tinctures. It is also used as a base for the Bach Flower Remedies, for the same reason.

Arab Medicine

While this generalized term is often misleading, it can fairly be applied to the period of Omayyad caliphs (Muslim rulers), who ruled during the first half of the eighth Christian century, when the empire extended from Spain to Samarkand. This was the beginning of an intense period of advancement in medical knowledge, made possible in large part by the translation of all the Greek medical writings into Arabic. A part of these historic labors was contained in the 400,000 volumes bound in leather and gold in the library of Hakim II of Spain. This activity reached its climax in the eighth century C.E. and lasted until the twelfth century. Eminent Arabic writers of the time included Hunain (809–873), Avenzoar (1113–1162), Rhazes (850–925), and, above all, Avicenna (980–1037). The latter, known as the Arabic Galen, and the Prince of Physicians, was a leading physician and scholar at the age of fourteen; his *Canon of Medicine* has been the most famous medical book in the history of the world.

Hunain's *Ten Treatises on the Eye* is the earliest systematic textbook on ophthalmology known, and Rhazes's "On Small Pox and Measles" gives the first clear account of these two diseases.

During these active centuries, the Arab Muslims made three fundamental contributions to medicine: the introduction of medicinal chemistry in the form of alchemy and botany, the organization of pharmacy, and the founding of hospitals. Muslim physicians and pharmacists were pioneers in chemistry and pharmacology; their extensive experimentation led to the development of the fundamental chemical processes of filtration, distillation, sublimation, and calcination. Geber distilled vinegar, sublimed sulphur, prepared sulphuric and nitric acids and mercury bichloride. Avicenna deduced the pharmacologic properties of herbs from their taste, color, and odor. Arabs experimented with their drugs on animals. The supervision of the pharmaceutical trade and licensing of physicians was devised by the Arabs.

There is little question that the Arabs significantly added to what was known of Greek medicine. This form of Arab medicine, called Tibb, was transmitted to Europe through Latin translations and today remains the primary mode of medical treatment for millions of persons in the Middle, Near, and Far East as well as parts of South America and Europe.

Acceptance of the Tibb-i-Unaani system seemed to falter for a time around the end of the eighteenth century C.E., but medical opinion is now changing and returning to it with new concepts in research and methodology. After the lapse of nearly two thousand years of medical study and experimentation in the doctrine of the humours, containing innumerable flirtations with hypotheses of disease, there is today a return to the original, perhaps ultimately indefinable notion of morbidity based on, and its varying manifestations colored by, the innate and vulnerable nature of the individual as a divine creation. (See also, *Tibb-i-Unaani, Avicenna.*)

Arnica *(Arnica montana)*

The plant used in herbal remedies is commonly called leopard's bane. Its medicinal properties are due to the alkaloid trimethylamine.

In small doses, it is a cardiac stimulant; in large doses, a depressant. The most popular application is the tincture or infusion applied externally in the treatment of sprains, bruises, abrasions, and similar surface wounds. *Taken internally, it frequently causes death.*

Aromatic Waters *(Aquae Aromaticae)*

Distilled water that is impregnated, often saturated, with a volatile substance, by (a) distillation—a heated mixture of drug or volatile oil with water, obtaining clear solution saturated with aromatic principle of plant; (b) solution—shaking occasionally during 12 hours, in large bottle, volatile oil .2 cc. with distilled water to make 100 cc., filtering to remove sediment; (c) aeration—passing gas into water.

An aromatic powder is made of 2 parts cinnamon, 2 parts ginger, 1 part cardamom, and 1 part nutmeg—all ground and sifted into a fine powder. Other common aromatics are anise, basil, black pepper, cajaput, caraway, cloves, coriander, dill, fennel, horehound, lemon peel, peach, peppermint, round pine, sassafras, valerian, vanilla, wild cherry, and wormwood.

Aromatics

Substances characterized by fragrant, spicy taste or odor such as cinnamon, ginger, the essential oils, and the like. They are generally stimulant to the mucous membranes of the gastrointestinal tract and are used as carminatives (agents that promote expulsion of gas) and as vehicles for administering nauseating remedies or drugs. In large doses, they irritate the stomach. *They should not be used in cases of inflammation of the stomach or bowels.*

Arrowroot *(Maranta arundinacea)*

A kind of starch derived from a plant native to the West Indies but also found in the southern United States. It is widely used as a food and is a popular remedy for diarrhea. The best variety comes from Bermuda. The arrowroot is best prepared by first mixing a small amount with milk into a smooth paste, thus avoiding lumps.

Asafetida *(Asafoetida Linné)*

Asafetida, also known as Food of the Gods and Devil's Dung, grows mainly in Afghanistan and eastern Iran. The chief uses for it are as a tincture, in pills, and in a mixture with magnesia as a remedy for flatulence. A gum resin obtained from the living root is a mild stimulant to the nervous system and the circulation. It is also used as an expectorant, a tonic, a laxative, a diuretic, an emmenagogue, an aphrodisiac, and an anthelmintic. The odor is extremely nauseating and persistent. It is used in suppository form for colic and gas in infants, in pill form for nervous diseases and hysteria.

Astringents

Agents that produce contraction of muscle fiber and condensation of other tissue, probably by direct irritation of the tissue and also by precipitating albumin and gelatin. The principal astringents are as follows:

acacia	dodder	male fern	shave grass
agrimony	echinacea	mullein	skullcap
azalea	elecampane	myrrh	squaw vine
barberry root	eyebright	olive	St. John's wort
betony	fumitory	periwinkle	strawberry
bistort	grape leaves	plantain	sumac
blackberry	hawthorne	pomegranate	uva-ursi
black cohosh	henna	quassia	wahoo
cassia	hops	quince	water plantain
cayenne	hydrangea	red raspberry	white pond lily
cinnamon bark	lobelia	red rose	yarrow
cloves	magnolia	sandalwood	yellow dock

and all teas with tannin.

Astrology

Mention of the stars in relation to physical, emotional, and mental health can be found as far back as the *Rig Vedas* (C. 1000 B.C.), the first religious texts in an Indo-European language. It was, however, Paracelsus, the sixteenth-century physician-astrologer, who related humans to the stars by means of the "sidereal body." *Sidereal* is a synonym for "astral," and denotes a kind of substance intelligible only to our "higher" sensitivities.

According to the yogic theories of the East, the ductless endocrine glands have been felt to be related to the various planets, or to be under their influence; that is, each organ is motivated and stimulated by a specific planet: the thyroid by the planet Mercury, the gonads by the planet Uranus, and so forth.

These concepts were added to and refined by Rodney Collins, the British disciple of Ouspensky, and the Italian Giordano Bruno. Bruno, who lived in the sixteenth century, introduced the idea that each individual is a *monad* which exists as a separate entity, while being aware of and permeated by the *monas monadum,* or world soul, which permeates everything.

Gottfried Wilhelm Leibniz (1646–1716) devised a "theory of reality" based upon the idea of the monad. In Leibniz's theory, monads have existed since the beginning of time, and are so closely interrelated that changes in one monad reflect the changes in another, or all other monads. It is these ideas of matter as force and man as a microcosm reflecting the forces of everything in the universe which form the basis of today's understanding of the relationship between stars and individual human acts.

Aura

The first attempt in this century physically to see the aura was in the early 1920s in London. Dr. Walter Kilner of St. Thomas Hospital developed a screen using a special dye which rendered the body's emanations visible.

The best-known researcher in the field of auras was Baron Karl von Reichenbach, a nineteenth-century biochemist who called these hues from the human body od, or odic force.

The aura is a visible sensation, like a gentle current of tinted air, rising from the limbs or body to the head. The problem is that not everyone is able to see auras, and while it is definitely necessary to "practice" identifying auras, sometimes even those who try for extended periods cannot become accomplished at this.

Auras are discussed in the writings of the earliest Christian mystics, and they are mentioned in virtually every other religious system. The representations of saints often include a halo, which is one type of aura.

The aura is usually divided into inner, outer, and middle sections and, when seen, occupies an area extending out from the body to about 1½ feet. Each of these layers has a different color, and those skilled at reading auras are able to construct elaborate diagrams and colored drawings of these auras, each of which is particular to an individual, like the uniqueness of a fingerprint.

Avicenna and *The Canon of Medicine*

Abu-Ali al-Husayn ibn Sina, known in the West as Avicenna, was one of the most illustrious physicians in recorded history. He was born in 980 A.D., near Bokhara in present-day Afghanistan. Though that was the center of learning of the time, he had exhausted all teachers of the day by the time he reached his teens, and was able to extend his logic teacher's understanding. He received no formal education in the sciences or medicine, but had physicians working under his direction when he was fourteen years old.

He is perhaps less known for his medical genius than for his philosophy. His book *Kitab-ul-Ansaaf* ("The Book of Impartial Judgment"), in which, at the age of twenty-one, he posed and answered twenty-eight thousand questions on theology and metaphysics—remains a significant and undisputed contribution to human thought.

Avicenna was extremely active in all realms of life, serving several times as a court minister and, on more than one occasion, being caught up in intrigues that led him to flight or to prison. He wrote whenever he could—in prison, on horseback, or in the wee hours of the night after working all day. He wrote in verse to instruct his pupils, and produced important works on Sufi doctrines and behavior. He never had a library and wrote primarily from memory. He is credited by scholars with an astounding outpouring of 276 works, touching on all aspects of human endeavor—medicine, natural history, physics, chemistry, astronomy, mathematics, music, economics, and moral and religious questions. Among them is one of the greatest classics on medicine, the eighteen-volume *Qanun-i Tebb* ("Canon of Medicine"), which covers and orders all the medical knowledge of the world up to his time. The *Qanun* maintained its authority throughout the world, and even today remains the bible of medicine for practitioners in India (both Muslim and Hindu) and throughout the Near and Middle East. Large medical schools are devoted to teaching Avicenna's methods, and in India, huge warehouse complexes are strategically located to supply the remedies from the *Qanun*.

Up to the end of the eighteenth century, the London Dispensary was considerably influenced by the herbal remedies of Avicenna, and their use continued widespread into the nineteenth century. In fact, many of his remedies are still used in western Europe and the United States, especially in rural areas that rely upon home remedies. It remains for Western medical science to study this rich source of knowledge as one of the greatest systems of empirical medicine ever devised.

Translations of Avicenna's *Qanun* remain incomplete and inadequate. A British doctor, Cameron Gruner, translated the first volume of the *Qanun* into English, having been introduced to Avicenna's work by Hazrat Inayat Khan, a Sufi mystic from Hyderabad, India. The remaining seventeen volumes are available in Persian and Arabic, with some translations into the Romance languages. (*See also Arab Medicine, Tibb-i Unaani.*)

Ayurveda

Ayurvedic medicine, based upon the "Theory of Tridoshas," is one of the oldest and noblest contributions of ancient India to world culture. Ayurvedic medicine has been known and practiced in India for over three thousand years, but its tenets are virtually unknown in the rest of the world.

The term *ayurveda* is composed of two Sanskrit words: *Ayu* meaning "life" and *ved* meaning "knowledge." Thus ayurvedic medicine is not simply a system for treating the ill, but a complete, rationalized system—sometimes called a "divine plan"—for maintaining the body in optimum mental, physical, and spiritual health, primarily by relying on preventive measures.

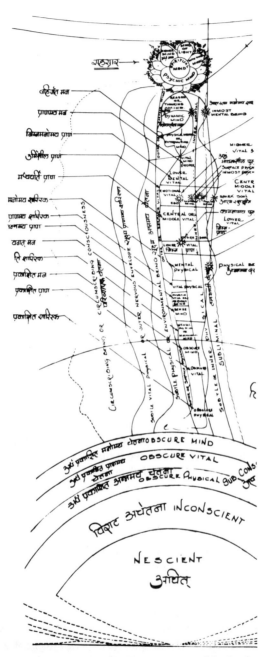

A schematic diagram of the divine plan of the body, according to which ayurvedic medicine is practiced. Drawn by Amidhar Bhatt of the Aurobino Ashram, this detailed illustration reveals the planes, parts, and entities of the total consciousness of a person.

Disease is avoided by following prescribed rules daily to promote active immunology and by attending to all of the body's natural functions. Humanity is divided into three groups, or *dhatas*—the Vata, the Pitha, and the Kapha—according to the dominance of one or more of the life processes, which are derived from one or more of the five "sheaths," or *pancha-koshas* (food, bio-energy, mind, intellect, and bliss eternal). The following are the basic daily rules for following the ayurvedic system of life:

1. Wake up early and go the the bathroom; wash the mouth and oral cavity.
2. Brush the teeth with fresh green twigs that are astringent, bitter, and pungent in taste.
3. Clean the tongue thoroughly with fingers and with the twig used like a brush.
4. Clean the eyes, ears, nose. Use hot water in the cold season, and cold water in the hot season.
5. Go in reverence and pay dutiful regards to parents and other elders in the family.
6. Put drops of oil in both nostrils and ears (better done at bedtime).
7. Eat *tambul (betel leaf)* as it cleanses the oral and facial passages of the mucous collected overnight.
8. Take an oil massage and bath. Rub the oil particularly well on the hands and soles of the feet, and also on the head and especially the crown.
9. Take regular exercise, but do not overdo this.
10. After breakfast proceed to your regular duties (trade, study, office work, etc.).
11. Eat lunch in a happy frame of mind. See that not only the elders, family servants, and others receive their quota of food, but also the family animals such as cows, sheep, dogs, etc.
12. Have a light evening meal and go to bed on a comfortable cot at an early hour.

A fine introductory text in English on ayurvedic medicine is *Ayurveda for Health and Long Life,* by Dr. R. K. Garde, available from D. B. Taraporevala Sons & Co., Private Ltd., 210 Dr. Dadabhai, Naoroji Road, Bombay 400 001, India.

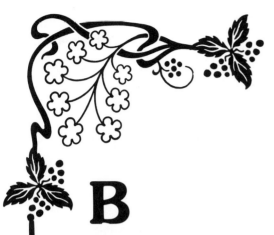

B

B Vitamins

When the B vitamins were first discovered, vitamins were identified by letter only; thus, vitamin B_1 was known as vitamin B; B_2 was vitamin G; B_6 was vitamin Y; biotin was vitamin H; and folic acid was vitamin M. Today, with new B-vitamin discoveries, the proper names of the identified elements are used instead.

B_1, now called *thiamine,* has the taste and odor of yeast and is destroyed rapidly by exposure to high, moist heat and alkaline solutions. Thus, boiling will destroy it. Whole grains, beef, nuts, liver, pork, and yeast are the foods containing the highest proportion of thiamine. The body can only store approximately a two-week supply. Eating large amounts of carbohydrates increases the need for thiamine. The minimum daily requirement is 1 milligram, which can be bought in synthesized form.

B_2, *riboflavin,* was discovered in connection with pellagra, a disease due to deficiency of niacin or nicotinic acid (B_3). When the niacin deficiency was corrected, there still remained a missing element, and vitamin B_2 was isolated. Evidences of riboflavin deficiency include sudden stoppage of growth, loss of hair, scaly skin, light sensitivity, and burning and red eyes.

Vitamin B_3, commonly called *nicotinic acid or niacin,* was also isolated in experiments relating to nutritional deficiency. Niacin is usually used as a superficial vasodilator, causing the blood vessels on the surface of the skin to dilate. The synthetic form of niacin, called niacinamide, is often used in place of niacin, usually to prevent the "flushing" and hot flashes so characteristic of niacin ingestion.

The richest sources of niacin are liver, lean meat, fish, wheat, legumes, and yeast. The minimum daily requirement for niacin has been established at 10 milligrams per day.

Vitamin B_6 is also called *pyridoxine* (vitamin Y according to the old terminology). Pyridoxine helps us determine whether things smell good or bad. For this reason, it is sometimes used in treating morning sickness in pregnancy. A little-known fact about pyridoxine is that it is necessary in the assimilation of melanin, which is essential for coloring the skin. Thus, some take pyridoxine to promote tanning in the sun. Pyridoxine is necessary for carbohydrate, fat, and amino-acid metabolism. Foods richest in pyridoxine are egg yolk, meat, fish, milk, whole grains, and cabbage. While a minimum daily requirement has not been established, most physicians recommend at least 10 milligrams per day to prevent deficiency.

Pantothenic acid, another of the B vitamins, is necessary for the assimilation of several other B vitamins, especially B_2. Sometimes called the antigray hair factor because of its ability to cure gray hair in rats, its use alone in humans does not produce the same effect. Pantothenic acid is necessary in metabolizing proteins, fats, and carbohydrates. Deficiencies of this vitamin may show as inflammation of the skin, spots on the cornea of the eye, fatigue, and numbness of extremities. Pigmentation of the skin is partially dependent upon pantothenic acid. About 9 milligrams of pantothenic acid are felt to be adequate, and deficiencies seldom occur due to the many foods in which it is readily available, including liver, eggs, kidney, beef, skim milk, buttermilk, molasses, peas, cabbage, broccoli, cauliflower, peanuts, sweet potatoes, kale, and yeast.

Vitamin B_{12}, called the antianemic vitamin, is unusual in that it is the only vitamin containing cobalt. At least 90 percent of B_{12} is destroyed as it passes through the stomach; thus it is usually given in therapeutic doses by injection. The main food source of B_{12} is liver, and it is usually not present in vegetarian diets, but is found in seaweed, some fermented soy products, comfrey, and egg yolk.

Biotin must be present in the body for beneficial bacteria to survive. Since the need for it is measured in micrograms, deficiency is quite rare. Biotin is involved in metabolizing fats—especially in depositing fat in the liver, in the form of cholesterol. Deficiency of biotin results in loss of hair, swelling and redness of the lips, and spots on the cornea of the eye. Raw egg white destroys biotin. Deficiency of biotin is easily prevented by addition of yeast to the diet.

PABA (para-aminobenzoic acid) is the other of the antigray vitamins, and is often taken with pantothenic acid to prevent graying of hair. Using it, the arctic explorer Adolphus Greely was successful in restoring his hair to blackness after an extended period of isolation and poor nutrition. However, it does not work alone, or for everybody, so there are other factors involved.

PABA reduces production of the thyroid hormone; thus those who take iodine or other substances designed to increase production of the thyroid must be careful of PABA consumption. PABA is present in large quantities in liver, yeast, rice, bran, and whole wheat. It is part of the folic-acid formula, so if one takes enough folic acid, one can be assured of taking enough PABA.

Folic acid is technically a group called folacin. It works with vitamin B_{12}, stimulating production of red blood cells, and is often used in treatment of anemia. Folic acid also works in conjunction with vitamin C. The name comes from the many plants whose "foliage" contains the folacin group. The best sources are yeast and cauliflower; meats contain very little. A 5-milligram tablet, by prescription, is a common dosage.

The Food and Drug Administration made folic acid a prescription item several years ago, and no more than .6 milligram can be included in over-the-counter preparations.

Non-B-Complex Vitamins

There are other recently discovered vitamins which are not usually placed directly in the B-complex group, but which, as therapeutic agents, are considered part of the group. One good example is *methionine,* which, as a food, is considered to be an amino acid; as a therapeutic agent, it is part of the B group. Choline and betaine are often listed with methionine and called lipotrophic agents (meaning that they assist assimilation of fats). *Pangamic acid* is often shown as vitamin B_{15}, and *laetrile* is called vitamin B_{17}. There remains debate as to whether these are definitely vitamins of the B group.

Alcohol is lethal to B vitamins in the body. Penicillin seems to destroy niacin. Generally speaking, blackstrap molasses, wheat germ, yeast, and yogurt included in the diet daily will supply the B-family vitamins in adequate quantities.

Bach Flower Remedies

Edward Bach (1886–1936) was born in London and trained at the University College Hospital there, qualifying for his doctor of medicine degree at age twenty-six. He operated his own clinic near the hospital for several years, until he became distressed at the serious side effects of chemical drugs. He thereafter applied his honesty and sincerity to a long research project which was aimed at determining how patients might best be treated. In this work, he was greatly influenced by Samuel Hahnemann's *Organon* (see *homeopathy*); from 1919 onward, the two men worked together as pathologists and bacteriologists at the London Homeopathic Hospital.

For his remedies, Bach turned to the nonpoisonous, harmless herbs, flowers, and twigs for bodily correction. He narrowed the remedies for all human complaints down to thirty-eight, which were prescribed entirely for mental symptoms without any regard for physical signs or symptoms.

Bach placed all human mental conditions into seven major classifications: fear, suffering incertainty, insufficient interest in present surroundings, loneliness, oversensitivity, despondency or despair, and overconcern for the welfare of others. He experimented widely on himself and devised a system for preparing the remedies which are used to this day.

The method requires obtaining the bloom or other part of the flower at its most "perfect" time of growth and placing the herb in pure spring water under direct sunlight for several hours. The "essence" thus extracted is then sensitized and diluted greatly and taken a few drops at a time with water.

Today the remedies are available from the Dr. Edward Bach Healing Centre in Mount Vernon, Sotwell, Wallingford, Berkshire, England. Some of the remedies, however, are made up and preserved in alcohol (often *saki*) a practice surely contraindicated by Bach.

The textbook for this system is *The Twelve Healers and Other Remedies,* by Edward Bach (London: C. W. Daniel, 1975).

Balm of Gilead *(Populus candicans)*

This tree is of the same species as the poplar and possesses some medicinal properties. The buds, bruised and tinctured in spirit, produce an effect similar to tincture of myrrh. It is taken internally as a restorative and externally for bathing sores. The bark, scraped from the twigs and steeped in hot water, is a good corrector of the bile and will operate as both an emetic and a cathartic. Due to the scarcity of this tree in its pure state in America, its use has been entirely replaced by the Balsam Fir.

Balmony *(Chelone glabra)*

Also called bitter herb, it grows wild in the United States in wet land. It is often cultivated for flowers in domestic gardens. Balmony is about the size of mint; the leaves are somewhat larger. It bears a white blossom of singular form, somewhat resembling a snake's head with mouth open. The leaves are dark green, with a sweetish bitter taste, and from this the name is derived, as the leaves are the medicinal part used. This herb is very good to correct bile, and it is the best herb available to improve appetite. A tea may be made using it alone or with other herbs calculated to restore the digestive powers. Some physicians also use it as an *anthelmintic*.

Balsam *(Abies balsamea)*

Balsams are volatile, resinous substances that contain benzoic, cinnamic, or similar acids. The principal balsams are those derived from Canadian fir. They are of a very healing nature and are good for removing internal soreness. Fir balsam is also used as a base in many healing salves. Taken orally, it is usually dropped onto a lump of sugar. It is expectorant and antiseptic and used in certain skin diseases.

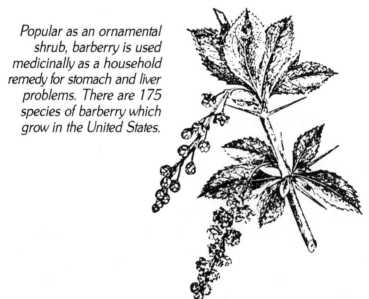

Popular as an ornamental shrub, barberry is used medicinally as a household remedy for stomach and liver problems. There are 175 species of barberry which grow in the United States.

Barberry *(Berberis vulgaris)*

The 175 species of this shrub make it a well-known and popular ornamental planting in the United States and Europe. It produces small clusters of yellow berries, which turn red when they ripen. In this condition, they are used for pickling and are also preserved with sugar and molasses. The bark of the root is used as a bitter to correct the bile and assist digestion. It has a folk medical history as a household remedy for stomach and liver problems. The berries are eaten raw for symptoms of typhus fever, and tinctures are applied in cases of female genital troubles, gall bladder problems, for increasing bile, and for reducing high blood pressure.

Barley-Water

A decoction of 2 ounces of barley boiled for 5 minutes in 1½ pints of water makes a nutritious demulcent drink in fevers and inflammatory conditions, especially when the gastric mucous membranes are inflamed.

Basal Metabolism

Basal metabolism is the caloric value which an individual produces while resting in bed and prior to taking breakfast; in other words, when the effects of food and exercise on caloric output are at a minimum. Basal metabolism is expressed in terms of calories per hour per square meter of body surface. It varies with age and is proportionate to body surface calculated from the height and weight of the individual. Metabolism usually should not vary more than 15 percent above or below normally accepted figures, which can be obtained from a physician, under whose direction the test must be given.

Bath

A medium in which the body is wholly or partly immersed. As therapeutic agents, baths are classified according to the form used, such as water, vapor, air, and so on, and according to the end desired: as nutritional, medicinal, stimulant. Among the special forms of baths are the Schott Treatment, Nauheim bath, electric light bath, sea-water bath, Russian bath, Turkish bath, sitz bath, and mud bath. (See also *Hydrotherapy.*)

Bayberry *(Myrica cerifera)*

Bayberry, also known as candleberry, is a species of myrtle growing in many parts of the United States. A shrub from 2 to 4 feet high, bayberry is recognized from its many waxy berries similar to juniper berries. The leaves are deep green. The bark of the roots is employed medicinally and should be collected in the spring before the leaf shoots appear or in the fall after growth has ended, as the sap is then collected in the roots (a general rule for collecting all roots for medicine).

Bayberry has been in use as a medicine since the time of Galen (third century A.D.) and is very stimulating and pungent, "prickling" the glands and causing the saliva and other juices to flow freely. It is also usefully employed as a tooth powder and most frequently used as a snuff to clear the nasal passages and for relief of headaches. It is employed as an emetic when the stomach is overfull, and as a cholagogue. The decoction is used on skin ulcers and all kinds of sores and carbuncles.

Bearberry *(Arctostàphylos Uva-Ursi)*

Also called mountain cranberry, it grows in dry, sandy soil in 3,000- to 9,000-foot altitudes in North America and south into Mexico. It produces urn-shaped white flowers tinged with red from June to September, and follows with red berries in the winter. The medicinal part is the green leaves, which are best picked and dried in autumn.

Bearberry is astringent, diuretic and tonic, and was used by the Indians to treat inflammations of the urinary tract, especially cystitis. It is almost legendary in the treatment of all urinary disorders, especially chronic afflictions of the kidneys, mucous discharge from the bladder, and urethritis. Combined with blueberry, it is helpful in treatment of diabetes. It is usually employed as a decoction and taken as a tea.

Belladonna (Deadly Nightshade) *Atropa belladonna*

The leaves and root of a European plant of the order of *Solanaceae*. The medicinal interest of Belladonna stems from two alkaloids it contains: atropine and belladonnine. The raw root and leaves are sometimes used medicinally in small doses.

Belladonna stimulates the heart and the vasomotor and respiratory systems and is used as a prescription drug in allopathic medicine to arrest secretions, relieve spasms, and dilate the pupils. It is also used to relieve pain from inflammation, cerebral and spinal congestion, inflammation of the lungs, iris, and bladder, cystitis, spasms, scarlet fever, and constipation. Locally applied, it is efficient in treating ulcers, fissures, boils, and abscesses. An extract can be prepared from the leaves, and it can be made into a tincture and an ointment. In cases of overdose or poisoning, opium is used as the physiological antagonist; tannic acid is the chemical antidote.

Belladonna is not usually available without a prescription, although it is an ingredient of some over-the-counter preparations, especially those of homeopathy. It is an extremely potent herb.

Benzoin (See also *Storax*)

A resin obtained from a tree of the genus *Styrax* native to Sumatra and Siam. It yields benzoic and cinnamic acid, is antiseptic and disinfectant, and is used primarily as a stimulating expectorant in chronic bronchitis. As a tincture, benzoin mixed with glycerin is favorably employed as a remedy for sore nipples during lactation; the compound tincture is inhaled as a sedative. Benzoin is also used as a cosmetic to remove freckles and for other skin conditions.

Bier's Hyperemic Treatment

The enforced flow of additional blood to an affected part of the body was developed by a German physician, August Bier (1861–1949). The part affected is placed in a specially constructed box, into which a current of hot air (144° to 230° F) is conducted through a tube. The degree of heat is not so high as to be painful; nor is it applied for more than one hour per day. Treatment should not be given during the menstrual period and is contraindicated in joint tuberculosis, as it provokes abscess formation.

Otherwise, the hypermic treatment is advocated for sciatica, lumbago, arthritis, varicose veins, and fractures. It is also claimed to be beneficial for gangrene, diabetes, and senility. There are also two "passive" forms of inducing blood flow—constriction and suction, produced by the elastic bandage and vacuum cup respectively. Careful and correct technique, applied by a skilled practitioner or physician, is requisite for the success of the treatment.

Bile

Bile is secreted by the liver. After bile is formed by the liver cells, it is transported from the liver to the gall bladder by the bile capillaries, which unite finally to form the main hepatic ducts.

Bile coming from the liver is primarily thin and watery. Bile obtained from the gall bladder is more or less viscous due to the presence of mucin. Bile is always alkaline when it is discharged from the liver, but it may become neutral in the gall bladder. When it is fresh, it has no odor, but it quickly breaks down and becomes offensive. The taste of bile is bitter. Bile obtained from the hepatic duct is variable in color; in humans, it is found to be both golden yellow and dark green, due to pigments.

In Eastern humoral medicine, there are felt to exist yellow and black bile, which form two of the four main components of the inner systems of "humours"of the body, the balance of which determines health (see *Tibb-i Unaani*). The composition of bile is:

water	977.40 Parts
sodium glycocholate	9.94
sodium taurocholate	trace
cholesterol	0.54
free fat	0.10
sodium palmitate and stearate	1.36
lecithin	0.24
organic matter and pigments	2.26
inorganic salts	8.36
	1,000.00 Parts

Biochemic Tissue Salts (See *Schuessler Tissue Salts*)

Birch *(Betula)*

The birch family is comprised of nearly forty species of trees and shrubs of the genus *Betula*. Birch are found in North America from the Arctic Circle to Texas and Florida. They are usually found in the woods, but they are also grown as an ornamental shrub throughout the United States. All parts of the leaves, buds, bark, and roots are used, and the applications are extensive. Among the better-known medicinal uses are those for diarrhea, dysentery, cholera, and all troubles of the alimentary tract. The cleansing properties of birch have been used successfully to treat rheumatism, dropsy, gout, and kidney and bladder stones. The charcoal is used for gas and indigestion, and the sap is used for anemia.

Blackberry *(Rubus fructicosus)*

The roots, leaves, and bark of *Rubus fructicosus* are all used medicinally. The blackberry has a root that lives for many years, producing fruit of black, juicy berries every other year. The vine dies back to the ground annually.

While it is primarily used as a food, the blackberry is an excellent astringent and tonic used in chronic diarrhea, dysentery and cholera. A decoction of the root, leaves, or both is consumed several times a day in cases of excessive menstruation and for fever. The leaves are bruised and applied locally for hemorrhoids.

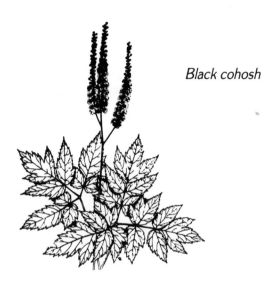

Black cohosh

Black Cohosh (*Cimicifuga racimosa*)

Also called squawroot and snakeroot, the plant is manifest in about twenty species in North America, Asia, and Europe. The most known in America are those of the "bugbane" variety, as they are used to drive away various insects. A tincture has been used externally by the Indians as an antidote for snakebite, and women have drunk black cohosh tea to relieve painful menstruation. It is used today in natural childbirth to speed contractions. Other applications, in tea decoctions and tincture, include those for high blood pressure, asthma, headache, migraine, female disorders, and as an expectorant.

Black Indian Hemp (See *Cannabis sativa*)

Bladder

This is the reservoir for the urine. A musculomembranous sac situated in the anterior portion of the pelvis behind the pubis, it is located in front of the rectum in the male and in front of the cervix uteri and vagina in the female. It is almost completely contained in the pelvic cavity, whether full or empty. Even distended, it may rise only slightly into the abdominal cavity. When moderately full, it measures about 3 inches by 5 inches and holds about a pint of fluid.

Urine is received from the ureters, which open into the bladder on the lower back side, and discharged periodically through the urethra. The ureters enter the bladder at an oblique angle, and there is a mucous membrane at each opening, which acts as a valve.

The urethra is the duct that carries the urine from the bladder to outside the body. In men, it also carries the seminal fluid. In women, its function is solely excretory.

Blass Oxygen Therapy

F. M. Eugene Blass, N.D., of New Jersey, died in October 1967 at the age of eighty-eight, as the result of a fall. He founded the Eastern American Association for Oxygen-Therapy, Inc., and held degrees in naturopathy, chiropractic, homeopathy, chemistry, and engineering, and was also a biologist and an oxidation specialist.

In 1922, he developed cancer of the pancreas. Through his knowledge in the engineering field, he developed Blass Oxygen Therapy to eliminate disease from humans and animals. His method consisted of cleansing the blood and vital organs through oxidizing the toxins and impurities in them, manipulation, hydrotherapy, and replenishing lacking minerals.

Blass's products—Magozone, Homozone, and Calozone—are made by a very complicated and time-consuming catalytic "ozonating" process, so that oxygen is bound to magnesium compounds (peroxide, hydroxide, and oxide), releasing about 6.7 percent active oxygen with Magozone and about 10 percent with Homozone, both having a laxative effect. With Calozone (which has an antilaxative effect), the active oxygen is bound to calcium. A mixture of Magozone and Calozone, named Macalozone, gives nearly normal stools. These minerals are thus carriers of vital nascent oxygen to the major fluid channels in the body, Blass contended, and thus throughout the whole body, thereby burning up the toxins and restoring normal oxidation and health to the body.

Blood, Chemical Analysis

The chemical analysis of blood is used in diagnosis, prognosis, and treatment of disease by medical doctors, naturopaths, and, in some states, chiropractors. It is particularly useful in diagnosing nephritis, diabetes, acidosis, comatose conditions, and gout, and in determining questions of kidney function.

The following table presents a summary of normal values of blood. The values are given in milligrams per 100 cubic centimeters of whole blood.

	Nonpro-tein Nitrogen	Urea Nitrogen	Uric Acid	Creatine	Sugar	Choles-trine	Chlorides	Plasma CO_2 capacity
Normal Blood	25–30	10–15	2–3	1–2	90–120	170–250	450–500	53–77

The *specific gravity* of blood varies from 1050 to 1060.

The *constituents* of blood are the plasma, red and white corpuscles, and platelets, fat globules, and other chemical substances.

The *red blood cells* carry oxygen and, in health, number from 4½ to 5 million to the cubic millimeter.

The *white blood cells* number from 7 to 9 thousand to the cubic millimeter. Varieties of white blood cells are large polynuclear, small mononuclear, transitional, eosinophil, and basophil.

The *blood platelets* number about 200,000 to the cubic millimeter.

Blood-Letting *(See Cupping, Leeching)*

Blood Pressure

The measurement of blood pressure, called sphygmomanometry, determines the amount of force necessary to equal the pressure in an artery in the extremities. For measurement, the brachial artery of the left arm is usually selected. An armband is applied to compress the blood vessels, and a bellows or pump is used to produce pneumatic pressure. A device (sphygmomanometer) to measure the amount of this pressure is also needed.

The following is the standard method of taking the blood pressure:
The cuff should be applied, preferably on the left arm, which should be level with the heart, the person sitting and the arm forward, unflexed and resting on a table. Place the stethoscope over the brachial artery, just below the sphygmomanometer cuff, and avoid undue pressure (evidenced by denting of the skin). Inflate the cuff until sound of the heartbeat cannot be heard through the stethoscope. Slowly release the air until the sounds reappear. The sound now heard is sharp and snappy, and is called the first phase, or *systolic pressure*. A succeeding sound, like a soft blowing murmur, is usually not recorded. A third

succeeding murmur is likewise not recorded. This muffled snappy sound continues for a varying number of beats and then becomes abruptly muffled. This is called the fourth phase, known as the *diastolic pressure.*

Blood pressure depends upon five factors: heart force, resistance, elasticity of blood vessel walls, amount of blood, and its viscosity. Systolic pressure represents the amount of force the heart uses to drive the blood through the arteries, while diastolic pressure represents the tension which the arterial walls exert upon the blood.

The *pulse pressure* is the difference between the systolic and diastolic pressures and is the energy of the heart which produces a distension of the arteries, simply called the pulse.

Blood pressure is influenced by many factors, some unrelated to health (blood pressure is lower in the morning than the afternoon, for example). A strong cup of coffee will raise the blood pressure approximately ten points, as will anger, passion, and muscular exercise.

The following is a table of normal pressures for children and adults. When giving the blood pressure, the systolic pressure is the one referred to, unless otherwise specified. This table shows systolic pressure.

Age	Male	Female
7	85	83
9	95	90
12	105	100
13	108	105
15	116	110
17	118	112
20 to 30	120–125	110–115
30 to 40	120–130	110–120
40 to 50	125–135	115–125
50 to 60	130–140	120–130
60 to 70	135–145	125–135
70 to 80	140–150	130–140

A safe but not infallible guide is that the pulse and the diastolic and systolic pressure should be in relation to each other as 1 : 2 : 3. Thus, an ideal ratio would be systolic 120, diastolic 80, pulse 40.

Blood pressure is increased in arteriosclerosis, toxemia, nephritis, nervous tension, and other diseases. It is lowered in general debility, anemia, low vitality, exhaustion, and heart failure.

Bloodroot *(Sanguinaria canadensis)*

A small herb, bloodroot is sometimes difficult to find in its native habitat under-growing forest trees. The fleshy root of the plant is quite brittle, and when it is broken, it exudes a red, "bloody" juice. The whole plant is medicinal, but mainly the root is used as a systemic emetic, an expectorant, an alterative, a tonic, a diuretic, and a febrifuge. In small doses, it stimulates the digestion; in large doses, it is an arterial sedative. Bloodroot excites the liver and is used as an enema for hemorrhoids, among other uses.
Bloodroot is often toxic in large doses.

Blood Wash

The blood-washing method, sometimes called the marathon bath, was invented by a Greek doctor named Christos Parasco in the 1800s. The wash consists of allowing a continuous shower of water at a temperature of 105 to 110 degrees to fall upon the body from a height of several feet. The subject lies under this stream for a period from two to eight hours, exposing different parts of the body to the shower from fifteen to thirty minutes each. The method is of value in weight reduction, but should not be used without careful supervision by those having high blood pressure, heart problems, or the aged. The blood-wash treatment is expensive, as it requires a continuous supply of water and the apparatus for heating it to the proper, controlled temperature. A substitute (for the debilitated, or for the sake of expense) is the "continuous tub bath," which can be borne for longer periods than the showers without causing weakness.

Blue Cohosh

Commonly called squawroot, squaw-weed, or blue or yellow ginseng, this tall perennial grows throughout the United States. The root and rhizome are most frequently used medicinally as an antispasmodic, a diaphoretic, or a parturient.

It is used in folk medicine for alleviating painful menstrual cramps and has gained fame for greatly alleviating—sometimes entirely—the pain of childbirth and for promoting prompt delivery. It is used as a tea in decoction during the last three to four weeks of pregnancy.

Other uses include applying as a poultice for skin sores, rash, and rheumatism, and as a tea in cold climates to warm the hands and feet.

Bodily systems

There are nine bodily systems as follows:
1. *The skeletal system:* all the bones of the body, known as the framework; held together by ligaments.
2. *The muscular system:* all the muscles of the skeleton, blood vessels, and hollow organs.
3. *The digestive system:* includes the teeth, salivary glands, esophagus, stomach, liver, gall bladder, pancreas, small intestine, and large intestine (colon).
4. *The respiratory system:* comprised of the nose, pharynx, larynx, trachea, bronchi, and lungs.
5. *The circulatory system:* the heart, blood vessels, lymphatics, blood and lymph.
6. *The exretory system:* the kidneys, ureters, bladder, urethra, skin, and lungs.
7. *The nervous system:* the brain, spinal cord, other nerves, and groups of plexii and ganglia.
8. *The reproductive system:* the testicles, vas deferens, seminal vessels, prostate, and urethra in the male; and vagina, uterus, ovaries, and fallopian tubes in the female.
9. *The endocrine system:* the thyroid, adrenals, thymus, pineal body, pituitary body, pancreas, part of the ovaries and of the testicles. The liver is also considered a gland of internal secretion.

Body, Chemical Elements in

The body is composed of the following chemical elements: carbon, hydrogen, oxygen, nitrogen, sulphur, phosphorus, fluorine, chlorine, iodine, silicon, sodium, potassium, calcium, magnesium, lithium, and iron.

Body, Daily Income and Output

Income	Grams	Output	Grams
protein	120	water	3,114.20
fat	90	urea	33.80
starch	330	salts	26.00
inorganic salts	32	extractives	6.00
water	2,818	feces	44.00
oxygen	744	carbon dioxide	910.00
TOTAL	4,134	TOTAL	4,134.00

Body, Bones in

The bones of the body are:

skull or cranium	8
face	14
small bones of ear	6
spinal column (including sacrum & coccyx)	26
ribs, sternum, and hyoid bone	26
upper extremities	64
lower extremities	62
TOTAL	206

Bougies, Pencils

Small solid cylinders of gelatin, glyco-gelatin mass (white gelatin 3 parts, glycerin 1 part), or oil of theobroma, impregnated with medicine, to be inserted into urethra, vagina, rectum, or nose.

Bouillon

An alimentary broth, made by boiling meat (usually beef) in water. Also, a liquid nutritive medium, made by boiling meat, for the culture of microorganisms. Solutions of bouillon can also be made from commercially-prepared powdered meats and used in special diets, for weight reduction, prevention of the loss of digestive power, and similar conditions.

Brain Extract

The extract of gray matter of the sheep's brain is sometimes used in general debility and in various nervous disorders and mental diseases. It is available commercially in tablet form in health-food stores or from a physician. A related substance, *cerebrin,* is an extract of ox brain.

Brand's Treatment

A fever treatment consisting of immersion in a cold bath of 68° F every three hours, or until the body temperature reaches 102° F. Friction massage is applied to the body while the temperature of the water is gradually reduced and cold is applied to the head. Stimulant drinks are administered after the bath, when the person is put to bed, warmly covered, and hot-water bottles applied to the feet.

The duration of the bath should be from five to fifteen minutes, ending sooner if the teeth begin to chatter and the lips turn blue. (See also *Cold, therapeutic.*)

Bread

A mixture of flour and water made porous by carbon dioxide and then baked. The flour may be of wheat, corn, oat, or rye. The carbon dioxide may be introduced by decomposing an alkaline carbonate (sodium or potassium), by an acid (cream of tartar), or by fermenting the starch with yeast.

Breast (See *Mammae*)

Broom *(Sarothamnus scoparius)*

The use of broom in medicine goes back to the Middle Ages, when it was employed by Welsh and Anglo-Saxon physicians. The tops of the brushlike branches are the part used in herbal medicine. Its properties are due to a neutral principle, scoparin, and an alkaloid, sparteine. In moderate doses, it is diuretic and laxative; in large doses, it is cathartic and emetic.

Broom tops are used as a tea in infusion and decoction, primarily for dropsy and kidney complaints. The dose of the fluidextract is ½ to 1 teaspoon, and of the infusion, 1 to 2 ounces.

Burdock *(Arctium lappa)*

Hunters know burdock from the pesky burrs which adhere to their clothing. Burdock was brought to the United States from Europe and grows wild on roadsides. The leaves of this plant, wilted by heat and applied to external injuries, will allay inflammation and ease pain. The leaves are also good when pounded and put on a bruise or sprain, and in case of fever to keep the feet moist and promote perspiration.

Burdock is used the world over as a blood-purifying agent as well as a diaphoretic, a diuretic, and an alterative.

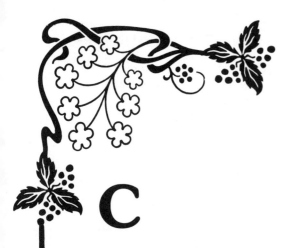

C

C Vitamin

Vitamin C is probably the best known and most widely used of the vitamins. It was first discovered when Jacques Cartier (1491–1557), a French explorer who opened up Newfoundland and Canada, connected scurvy with the absence of fresh fruit and vegetables. This discovery was made during a voyage in 1534.

Ascorbic acid, a synthetic form of vitamin C, does not appear in nature, and thus a slight controversy has sprung up over which form is to be preferred. The best nutritional physicians feel that ascorbic acid (synthetically made and less expensive) will work as well as vitamin C when the purpose of the use is as an antibacterial agent. For simple nutritional use, the true vitamin is preferred.

Literature on vitamin C is extensive; it has been claimed to have a therapeutic effect on everything from colds to cancer.

Vitamin C is soluble in water and insoluble in oil; thus, it must be taken with water to be assimilated. Vitamin C is destroyed by alkalies, and by drying of the fruits or vegetables containing the vitamin. Freezing, however, has no effect on it.

Vitamin C cannot be stored in the body; test animals deprived of vitamin C in their diets begin to show signs of deficiency within two weeks. A daily supply of vitamin C is recommended. Deficiency signs in humans include swelling and tenderness of the joints, appearance of nodules on the rib cage at the juncture with the sternum, bleeding of gums or loosening of teeth, slow healing of wounds, and inability to metabolize amino acids.

Since each person's requirements are different, a "threshold test" has been developed which measures the amount of vitamin C "spilling over" into the urine.

Requirements for vitamin C are felt to increase during pregnancy, infectious diseases, gastrointestinal problems, endocrine disturbances, and malignancies.

The minimum daily requirement established for vitamin C is 30 milligrams per day, although some physicians recommend doses of up to 1,000 milligrams per hour and even higher for specific diseases and therapeutic diets.

It is estimated that each cigarette smoked burns up 25 milligrams of vitamin C. Foods high in vitamin C include all citrus fruits, green peppers, spinach, parsley, tomatoes, liver, and milk.

Cacao Butter *(Oleum theobromatis)*

A fixed oil expressed from the seeds of the chocolate tree *(Theobroma cacao)*, it is a yellowish-white solid of faint odor, bland taste, and neutral reaction. Its action is demulcent, and it does not become rancid upon exposure to air. Its chief uses are in making skin-protection creams and oils and suppositories.

Cachets *(de pain)*, Konseals, Wafers

Various-sized concave wafers made of unleavened bread (flour and water) or wafer paper, which contain a drug within a cavity formed by moistening the concave edges of two and pressing together. When fastened, they are floated in water and gulped down.

Caffeine

This alkaloid is obtained from the leaves and seeds of the *Coffea arabica* or coffee plant and from the dry leaves of *Thea sinensis.* When it is extracted, the alkaloid appears as long, silky needles. A rapidly acting stimulant to the heart, brain, spinal cord, muscles, respiratory system, and kidneys, caffeine is consumed by the majority of adult Americans in coffee beverages and is used therapeutically in enemas as a part of detoxification programs. As an extracted drug, it is used as a stimulant in various poisonings and in combination with coal – tar drugs to combat their depressing action.

Cajuput Oil

A volatile oil distilled from the leaves of *Melaleuca leucadendron,* its action is similar to that of turpentine. It is used to relieve toothache and to treat skin disorders, flatulence, colic, dropsy, and hysteria.

Calamus (Sweet Flag) *Acorus calamus*

The rhizome of calamus contains a volatile oil and bitter principle and is used as an aromatic and a stomach tonic, usually in a fluidextract.

The rhizome from India is felt to be the best, although it is indigenous to the northeastern United States. Its use is recorded in the Bible in connection with dyspepsia and bronchitis.

Calcium

The most abundant mineral in the body, calcium is a silver-white metal characterized by a strong affinity for oxygen. Calcium constitutes more than one-half the mineral matter of the body. Calcium must be dissolved by an acid, and thus the absorption of it into the body, despite large intake, is often low.

Signs of calcium deficiency include poor blood clotting, muscle cramps, rapid pulse, and rapid breathing.

The ideal amount of calcium in the bloodstream is between 900 and 1,100 grams per 100 millimeters; a ratio of 10:1 is ideal.

The adult daily requirement of calcium is 750 milligrams per day—the highest requirement established for any vitamin or mineral.

The three main forms of calcium for nutritional use are calcium lactate, calcium carbonate, and calcium gluconate. Calcium lactate is the most easily assimilated. Food sources are oyster shell, eggshell, bone meal, and dolomite—although none of these sources is assimilated well into the body. Milk is perhaps the best source, as it is assimilated well.

It is felt that vitamin D is necessary for, or at least improves, the absorption of calcium from the intestines.

Calcium is also known in the form of an oxide, or quicklime, and a carbonate, called chalk. It is used medicinally in various ways, including application for burns and scalds, as a mouthwash, an antiseptic, a disinfectant, in inhalations, and for diarrhea.

Many herbs contain calcium, a general rule being the darker the leaf, the more calcium it contains.

Calendula *(Calendula officinalis)*

Among the many flowering garden varieties of marigold, only the deep, orange-flowered variety has medicinal value. Calendula is chiefly used as a local remedy, made into a tincture and applied to bruises, sprains, muscle spasms, ulcers, and similar problems.

Calendula officinalis can also be applied to bee and wasp stings and can be used as a tea for fevers and as a snuff to discharge mucus from the nose.

Calumba *(Jateorhiza palmata)*

One of the purest bitters known is derived from the root of this climbing plant, native to South Africa and the East Indies. It contains the alkaloid *berberine* and a bitter principle, *calumbin.*

It is usually given as a cold infusion to tone the gastrointestinal tract, for fevers, and diarrhea. In Africa and the East Indies, it is cultivated for use as a clothing dye.

Camphor

A ketone obtained from *Cinnamonum camphora,* a tree indigenous to eastern Asia. Camphor yields *camphoric* and *camphoretic acids,* has a hot, acrid taste, and is irritating to the mucous membranes. In large doses, camphor depresses the heart, lowers blood pressure, slows reflexes, and sometimes produces coma and death. (The poisoning is treated by coffee, emetics, and stimulants.)

Camphor is used in various forms of diarrhea to sedate the nerves, as a liniment for sore muscles, in vomiting, and for whooping cough, hysteria, and epilepsy. In the East, it is also used as a preservative for bodies of the deceased.

Cannabis

Known as hemp, Indian hemp, hashish, bhang, gunjah, dope, pot, and many other names, it contains cannabinone, cannabene and the hydride of cannabene. It is hypnotic, antispasmodic, diuretic, anesthetic, expectorant, aphrodisiac, cathartic, and tonic. In large doses, it produces mental exaltation, intoxication, and a sensation of double consciousness. It is consumed alone, as a rolled cigarette, in tea, and other ways by a substantial portion of the population (especially since the Vietnam War) as a relief from anxiety, for psychological excitation, and for other reasons. Medically, it has been used since the mid-1800s, and recently has been revived for treating glaucoma and to alleviate the pain of X-ray treatments for various degenerative diseases. Its folk-remedy applications include worms, catarrh, diabetes, diarrhea, dropsy, hydrocephalus, nausea, neuralgia, and vomiting.

Cantharis

Spanish fly, or cantharis, is extracted from the dried body of a species of beetle, *Lytta vesicatoria*. Locally applied, cantharis is a rubefacient and vesicant; internally it is an irritant, causing vomiting.

The tincture has been used internally in amenorrhea, in the later stages of nephritis from alcoholism, and for sexual impotency. In small doses, it has been used locally for psoriasis, eczema, and seborrhea.

Capsules

Various-sized transparent casings (short tubes, usually with one open end fitting over that of another) of hard or soft gelatin for administering nauseous or disagreeable liquids or solids.

Carbohydrates

One of the six elements of consumable foodstuffs, carbohydrates technically include starches, gums, sugars, and dextrins. Approximately one-half of all food intake is in the form of carbohydrates. The most basic carbohydrate is sugar, or refined sucrose, the main energy fuel utilized by the body. The blood sugar level is affected by intake and assimilation of carbohydrates; unbalanced sugar level leads to conditions such as hypoglycemia and diabetes. Excess sugar in the blood is known to cause diabetes, and too little blood sugar results in symptoms of mental confusion, procrastination, lack of drive, and similar states.

In the process of converting carbohydrates into forms usable by the body, calcium, magnesium, and other substances must be present. 80 percent of the energy that comes from blood sugar is expended to maintain the body temperature, and 20 percent goes toward calorie expenditure.

Practically all vegetables contain some carbohydrates. Overconsumption of starchy carbohydrates produces a tendency to flatulence, digestive disorders, constipation, enlarged tonsils, and other ailments. Those containing the least amount of starchy carbohydrates are:

Green beans	green peas	dandelion greens
cabbage	lettuce	radishes
cauliflower	celery	parsley
asparagus	onions	spinach
endive	beet tops	

The typical diet contains more starch than is required by the body. The starchy carbohydrates are:

cane sugar	dates	grapes
honey	figs	apples
syrups	maple sugar	bananas
		all other sweet fruit

Cardamom *(Elettaria cardamomum)*

The fruit of *Cardamom,* cultivated in Malabar, is a seedpod which is an aromatic, a carminative, and a stomachic. The seeds are about a fifth of an inch long, angular, wrinkled, and whitish. When they are powdered, they should be used immediately, as the powder loses its aromatic properties quickly.

Cardamom is used as a spice in foods and desserts, is added to tea, and is chewed with betel nuts in India. The main medicinal use is for indigestion. Adulterations include orange seeds and unroasted coffee grains.

Cardiants

Remedies that affect the heart, cardiants are either sedatives, stimulants, or tonics. *Sedatives* lessen the force and frequency of the heart's action. The most commonly used are aconite, antimony, cold temperature, digitalis, and senega. *Stimulants* rapidly increase the force and freqency of the pulse in depressed conditions of the heart muscle. Often-used stimulants are alcohol, aromatic oils, camphor, cayenne, cocaine, counterirritation, galvanic current, heat, spearmint, and turpentine. *Tonics,* when given in moderate doses, stimulate the cardiac muscles, slowing and strengthening their contractions. The chief tonics are caffeine, convallaria, digitalis, hellebore, and valerian.

Carminatives

Herbs or substances that aid the expulsion of gas from the stomach and intestines by stimulating peristalsis, stimulating the circulation, and relaxing the cardiac and pyloric orifices of the stomach, carminatives also act as diffuse stimulants of both bodily and mental faculties.

The principal carminatives are asafetida, camphor, horseradish, cayenne, cardamom, fennel, ginger, mace, mustard, pepper, prepared spirits; oils of: anise, cajuput, caraway, cinnamon, cloves, coriander, eucalyptus, fennel, nutmeg, peppermint, pimento, spearmint, and valerian root.

Cascara Sagrada *(Rhamnus purshiana)*

Rhamnus purshiana is also known as California buckthorn. The bark of a California plant, its medicinal properties are due to a volatile oil. Usually used as a fluidextract, it acts as a tonic to the intestines as well as a laxative. It is said that secondary constipation, which is so common with other laxatives and purges, does not occur with cascara sagrada. It has a very bitter taste, which can be masked by adding syrup of orange; best taken at bedtime.

Cassia (See *Cinnamon*)

Cassia Fistula

The pulp of a tropical fruit, *purging cassia,* as it is also known, is given as a laxative and cholagogue and is an ingredient in the confection made from senna.

Castor Oil

A fixed oil expressed from the seeds of *Ricinus communis,* castor oil is one of the best simple, nonirritating purgatives or cathartics. It is also used in the manufacture of soaps. The leaves, applied locally, have galactagogue properties. The taste of the oil may be disguised by adding a little oil of apricot kernels, coffee, orange juice, and the like.

Cataplasms, Poultices

Soft, pasty masses to supply moisture and warmth locally in order to break down inflamed tissue; flaxseed meal, slippery elm, hop, bread and milk, kaolin and glycerin, bran, and oatmeal work well for these, to which either tincture of aconite or arnica may be added to lessen pain. The true poultice should be made by bringing the mass, moistened with water or milk, to a boil, enclosing it in a cheesecloth bag, and applying it ½- to 1-inch thick over inflamed area. The addition of a little fixed oil or glycerin serves to retain heat and prevent caking, while a covering of oiled silk retains these properties much longer.

Catarrh

Inflammation of any mucous membranes, especially those of the nose.

Cathartics (Purgatives)

Agents that increase or hasten intestinal evacuation. *Laxatives* are nonirritating and excite moderate peristaltic action. The principal herbs of this class are cassia, manna, tamarind, cascara sagrada, and coffee.

Simple puragatives produce free discharge from the bowels, with some irritation and cramping. These enclude aloes, calomel, castor oil, rhubarb, and senna.

Drastic purgatives produce violent action of the bowels, with much irritation, pain, and spasms. Some of these are colocynth, croton oil, gamboge, jalap, and scammony.

Catheter

A tubelike instrument for evacuating the liquid contents of a cavity, usually the bladder. Catheters are made of soft rubber, woven silk, silver, or celluloid. The various diameters and lengths are suited to specific cavities, sex, age, and so forth.

Catnip

In addition to its fame as an excitatory agent for cats, catnip, a perennial herb found throughout the United States, is also used medicinally as an antispasmodic and a carminative, a stimulant, a tonic, a diaphoretic, an emmenagogue, and a fertility agent.

Cayenne *(Capsicum frutescens)*

Cayenne was brought to England from India in 1548, and its use was recorded in the Edinburgh Dispensatory until the middle of the eighteenth century. It gained wide fame in the United States—which continues to this day—when its medicinal use was discovered, quite accidentally, by Samuel Thomson, the unorthodox nature healer of New England. The word *cayenne* comes from the Greek "to bite," and despite the sharp stinging taste, it is used for a very long list of ailments.

Cayenne contains capsicin (a red coloring matter), oleic, palmitic, and stearic acids; its medicinal effect, which seems chiefly beneficial, occurs through its action as a catalyst for speeding other ingredients quickly throughout the body. Samuel Thomson used cayenne to promote and continue the internal combustive heat produced by lobelia, and it is always recommended to take the two together.

In the past, it was erroneously claimed that cayenne would cause injury by burning the stomach, but popular use has proved that it has successfully healed stomach ulcers and is one of the most powerful stimulants known among herbs.

The preparation includes grinding the pepper (African Bird Pepper is the best kind) into a fine powder. A dose is from ½ to 1 teaspoonful in hot water. All herb books contain dozens of applications for cayenne.

It is sometimes adulterated with salt, sawdust, and other substances, so purity must be determined to insure effective action.

Cells, of the Body

The human body is composed of masses of single structures called cells. These have different sizes, shapes, chemical compositions, and functions, and are grouped together to form different tissues, organs, and organ systems.

The cell is an organized mass of jellylike, colorless material called protoplasm; the body of the cell is called the cytoplasm, and within the center of the cell is a nucleus. Within the nucleus is a still smaller center, called a nucleolus. Within the cell also is a minute protoplasmic body called the centrosome, which regulates cell division.

Each live cell has five functions: *Irritability:* a live cell receives stimuli and therefore possesses irritability, though some cells are more sensitive to stimuli than others. The skin of the fingertips contains this type of cells. *Conductivity:*

any stimulus received by a cell results in a characteristic response, which is then conducted to other cells. The nerve cells possess this quality to a high degree. *Contractility:* the protoplasm has the power to contract, shown in the muscle cells. *Metabolism:* each cell has the means to maintain life by selecting nutritive building material from its environment—the blood and lymph. This process is called anabolism; the removal of the by-products of this process of sustaining life is called metabolism. The cells of the digestive tract possess the power of metabolism to a marked degree. *Reproduction:* the creation of a new human individual is the role of specialized sex cells, although some other cells (such as those of the skin) also have the ability to reproduce.

The organization by structure and function of cells in turn provides masses of cells in tissues and organs, which make up the various systems of the body.

Chalk

Prepared chalk is a native calcium carbonate, white and powdery, odorless and tasteless, insoluble in water. It is used as a mild astringent and antacid, as a tooth powder and dusting powder.

Chamomile *(Matricaria chamomilla)*

An infusion of the small flower heads acts as a tonic, digestive aid, and calmative, while in large doses, it acts as an emetic and a diaphoretic. It is applied locally in compresses and packs to relieve pain of sprains and bruises. The oil is quite useful in spasm relief, hysteria, asthma, and diarrhea.

It is a very widely known and used herb, especially for children, and a small cup of tea will enhance perspiration and elimination. The best chamomile comes from southern Europe.

Chaparral *(Larrea tridentata)*

The leaves and stems of chaparral, also known as creosote bush or greaseuoral, contain many gums, resins, acids, small amounts of a mixture of sterols; sucrose, protein, alcohol, and very little volatile oils. Chaparral is nontoxic and contains no alkaloids.

Its use among the Indians of the United States and Mexico has been widespread, and a plant with similar qualities is found in northern Argentina. Chaparral is antiseptic, diuretic, expectorant and tonic.

The plant has become popular in the past few years as a treatment, or part of a treatment, for cancer and other degenerative diseases. It is thought to be especially able to reorient the body's fermentation process by means of an active ingredient known as nordihydroguiaretic acid (NDGA). Several magazines have reported remissions and shrinkage of tumors with treatment consisting only of chaparral tea.

Chaparral is also used externally as a poultice for rheumatism and sprains, and its leaf residue—what is left after commercial processing for the resins—is fed to livestock, for it contains as much protein as alfalfa.

Charcoal

Charcoal exists in two forms: animal charcoal, prepared from bone in powder form, which is tasteless and odorless; and vegetable charcoal, prepared from soft wood and being very finely powdered, black, and shiny, which is also without odor or taste.

Charcoal is mainly used as an absorbent for foul gases, as a deodorant and as a disinfectant. It is used internally for flatulence and excess acidity, in chronic gastric catarrh, cancer, diarrhea, intestinal flu, and as a disinfectant for poisoning.

Charta

Papers coated or saturated with some medicinal substance, to be used as a plaster or for burning.

Cherry Bark *(Prunus virginiana)*

The young, thin bark of the cherry tree is native American—as nearly everyone who has even taken cough medicine knows—and is what gives most syrups their characteristic sweet cherry flavor. However, the cherry bark is healing in its own right, and has been applied for a wide range of afflictions from diarrhea in children, hectic fever, scrofula, and bronchitis to heart palpitation and indigestion.

Chicory Root *(Cichorium intybus)*

Commonly called endive or garden chicory, the root of chicory is consumed by many people daily, as the roasted root is used as an adulteration in many coffees. It is the chicory root which gives coffee its deep, rich brown color and somewhat bitter taste, and also slightly offsets the extreme excitability caused by caffeine.

Its medicinal action is hepatic, laxative, diuretic, and tonic, and it has been used for centuries in the East as a restorative herbal tea for liver complaints. The leaves can be eaten in salads, although they should be blanched slightly to lessen their bitter taste.

Chicory tea helps remove phlegm, especially from the stomach or colon if taken by enema. It is used medically in tincture form to sedate the central nervous system and for heart conditions.

Chiropody (Podiatry)

Chiropody is that healing art which specializes in treatment of the feet. Since a total of twenty-six bones are located in the feet, as well as many muscle groups in which practically all the nerves of the body have endings, the feet are felt to reflect and influence the health of the entire nervous system and body. Ill-fitting shoes, boots, and high-heeled shoes are felt to create the discomforts and misalignments of the feet and reflect, or sometimes cause, illness. The chiropodist uses various mechanical devices to balance the feet and correct problems, and sometimes performs minor surgery. Massage of the feet is employed to relax muscles in spasm, and a system of organ correspondences has been worked out to assist in pinpointing trouble areas in related parts of the body (see *Reflexology*).

Chiropractic

The origin of the science of chiropractic is credited to Daniel David Palmer (1845–1913), who, in 1895, succeeded in curing a man's deafness by adjusting his back following a strain suffered while working in tight quarters. Palmer examined the man's back and found one of the vertebrae badly out of alignment with the rest of the spine. Using his "instinct," Palmer gave a spontaneous "thrust" to the vertebra, and shortly thereafter, the man regained his hearing.

Following this coincidental cure, Palmer immersed himself in the study of anatomy and physiology, and after a great many similar successes on new patients, set forth the Principles of Chiropractic. These principles remain the basis of that science today, although chiropractic has undergone many refinements and advances.

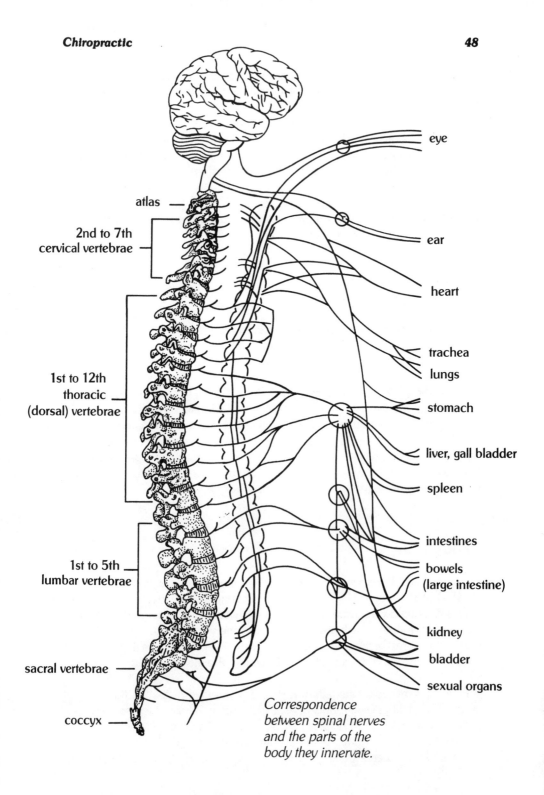

Correspondence between spinal nerves and the parts of the body they innervate.

Palmer posited that nerve impulses flowing through normal channels produce normal physiological functions. Any interruption or limiting of such free flow of nerve impulses results in reduction or alteration of corresponding organ functions. Among the forces that alter nerve flow, Palmer believed, were irritation of the nerves themselves, muscle spasms, and the resulting displacement of spinal processes. The chart below gives the placement of the nerves along the spine, and the corresponding areas they affect in the body.

The researches of Palmer were carried on by his son, Bartlett Joshua Palmer, and his father's colleague, Willard Carver. The Palmer College of Chiropractic today is considered one of the finest in the United States.

Many chiropractors utilize allied health sciences such as iridology, applied kinesiology, and dietetics as part of a full, "natural healing," clinical approach to health, with vitamin therapy a prominent feature among their recommendations. The displacement of vertebrae is determined by X-rays of the spine and various chemical tests including those of blood, urine, and biochemical assay.

While chiropractic was persecuted in its early stages by orthodox medicine and the practitioners labeled in derogatory ways, it has today become a full-fledged science, with chiropractic physicians having full licensing protection by state law.

Following are some of the ailments that have responded successfully to chiropractic techniques: arthritic pains, bursitis, disc syndromes, myositis, neuralgia, posture defects, lower back pain, sciatica, athletic injuries, sprains and strains, headaches, high blood pressure, nutritional deficiency, and related problems.

Chloride

Chloride, the ion of the chlorine atom, is highly soluble in water and rapidly disperses throughout the body's cell membranes. Its function is to maintain a normal electrolyte balance in tissues and normal osmotic pressure of body fluids. Nearly all plants and green vegetables contain substantial amounts of chloride, so deficiency is uncommon. Excessive amounts cause vitamin E to be destroyed and reduce the production of iodine. Foods rich in chloride are milk, radishes, olives, figs, kelp, and cheese.

Chlorides

Chlorides are derived from foods that have not been utilized by tissues, and are detected and measured as one of the constituents of urine. Persons in normal health pass from 10 to 15 grams per day, although this amount varies according to intake of salt. The excretion of sodium chlorides in urine is reduced in fevers, pneumonia, nephritis, diarrhea, anemia, and during sleep. Retention of chlorides in the blood and tissues results in excessive water retention in the tissues, causing edema.

Cholagogues

These are agents that stimulate the flow of bile and produce purgation at the same time. Among the primary cholagogues are aloe, bayberry, beets, cassia fistula, dandelion, fennel, gentian, golden seal, hops, jalap, manna, rhubarb, stillingia, wahoo, and wood betony.

Chromotherapy (Color Therapy)

The German optician Josef von Fraunhofer (1787–1826) developed an analysis of the color spectrum, a series of images appearing as narrow bands of color with a beam of light. The rainbow is a color spectrum.

The application of healing methods using the color spectrum borrows from astronomy, astrophysics, and even naval navigation (the "ring around the moon" phenomenon and ice crystals in cirrostratus clouds are examples of solid substances which produce a spectrum). Some hospitals and offices employ consulting agencies to advise on which colors have the best psychological effect in particular situations. Healers have worked with color for millennia. One analysis of the therapeutic action of colors follows:

> A true *green* soothes and quiets the nervous system, easing circulatory and heart ailments.
> Having a stimulating effect upon the nerves and blood, the color *red* is of value in treatment of anemia, paralysis, tuberculosis, physical exhaustion, and debilitation of the body. Not advised for fever conditions or inflammatory and nervous troubles.
> *Reddish orange* is felt to be beneficial for treatment of cancerous and malignant growths.
> *Yellow* affects the liver, digestive problems, and some eye and throat ailments.
> *Orange* benefits digestive and colonic disturbances, constipation, female pelvic disorders, and hernia.

Blue and violet are sedative and astringent, are quieting and soothing to the nervous and vascular systems, and are used in diseases such as neuralgia, rheumatism, hemorrhage, and sciatica; to stimulate the pineal body, and to ease pain of childbirth.

Cinchona Bark *(Cinchona officinalis)*

Also known as Peruvian bark, this is the bark of several varieties of cinchona, a tree native to the eastern slopes of the Andes. Cinchona bark contains twenty-four alkaloids, one of which is quinine, which accounts for most of its physiological and therapeutic actions. It is astringent, bitter, and tonic, and is used successfully in the treatment of malaria in all parts of the world, principally as a fluidextract or tincture.

Cinnamon *(Cinnamomum cassia)*

The common synonym for cinnamon is Annam cassia, sometimes shortened to cassia, after the province in China to which it is native.

The plant is a handsome evergreen tree, growing to a height of 20 to 30 feet. Cinnamon was a very early favorite spice, being brought by Arabian navigators to the Phoenicians, Greeks, and Romans. While there are some fifty species that grow wild, only a few yield the commercial bark, which today results mostly from commercially cultivated plants.

The constituents are a volatile oil (about 2 percent), tannin (up to 5 percent), resin, bitter principle, sugar, mannite, starch, mucilage, and ash.

Its medicinal properties are carminative, stomachic, stimulant, astringent, hemostatic, aromatic, antispasmodic, and germicidal. A volatile oil of cinnamon is distilled from the leaves, twigs, and waste bark and rectified by steam distillation. While the oil has no astringency, it is common as a household remedy for toothache. It is also used to treat diarrhea, flatulence, nausea, vomiting, menorrhagia, as a parturient, and also for flavoring bitter preparations and in the manufacture of chocolate. Dosage of the oil is 1 to 3 drops in a glass of water. A tea is often made from chips of the bark for digestive correction.

Citric Acid

Occurring freely in lemons, black currants, beets, and various acid fruits, it is a refrigerant, an antiseptic, and a diuretic.

Clove *(Eugenia aromatica)*

The unexpanded flowers of cloves are distinguished by their pungent, spicy taste. Its properties are due to a volatile oil, which is an antiseptic, an expectorant, a stimulant, and an irritant. Clove is given in powdered form for nausea, flatulence, and to aid digestion. The oil is used as a stimulant for peristalsis and as a feeble local anesthetic for decayed and painful teeth.

Clyster (See *Enema*)

Cocaine

The chief alkaloid extracted from *Erythroxylon coca,* its first action is as a stimulant to the respiratory and circulatory organs and to the nerve centers. In large, extended dosages, it is narcotic and depressant. One habituated to cocaine may suffer insomnia, decay of intellectual vigor, coma, and death. With small, repeated doses, side effects include vertigo, nausea, difficult articulation, restlessness, and heat flushes.

Cocaine is used medicinally as an anesthetic for minor surgery of the nasal passages and as an ingredient in many other topical anesthetics.

It has become a recreational drug for a portion of the American public, with approximately 25 percent of persons over age fifteen having experimented with it. The extreme cost for use of even small amounts prohibits its recommendation.

Cod Liver Oil *(Oleum morrhuae)*

The fixed oil obtained from fresh livers of the *Gadus morrhua* and other species of codfish, it contains bromine, iodine, sulphuric and phosphoric acids, and foreign material. It has tonic and alterative properties and contains large amounts of vitamins A and D. It is taken in capsule and emulsion form when malnutrition and lowered digestive vitality are present (for example, in scrofula, syphilis, rickets, sciatica, lumbago, neuralgia, and emphysema). It has a very bitter taste, which is masked by various substances such as glycerin, the aromatic oils of orange, lemon juice, and coffee.

Colchicum (Meadow Saffron) *Colchicum autumnale*

The root and seed of this plant have been used medicinally by the Arabs as a successful agent to relieve gout. The action is caused by an alkaloid called colchicine, which, besides being an emetic, a diuretic, a diaphoretic, and a drastic cathartic, may cause severe mental depression and has caused death by poisoning.

Cold, Therapeutic

Depending on the manner of application, cold is anesthetic, antiphlogistic, antiseptic, hemostatic, or tonic in action. Equal amounts of ice and salt, or plain ice in rubber bags or bladders, are often applied to head injuries, swollen joints, sprains, neuralgia, fever, and other ailments. Cold enemas are useful for bleeding hemorrhoids, dysentery, pruritis, bleeding from the vagina, and reduction of temperature. *Cold baths* have tonic and antipyretic effects. Hip baths of cold water are employed in pelvic weakness and hemorrhoids. The cold pack is valuable to reduce temperature: the person is wrapped in a sheet which has been soaked in ice water and wrung out. As it warms, it is replaced by a fresh cold one (ice water may be poured on) or lumps of ice are placed around it. When the patient's temperature is reduced, the sheet should be removed and a light blanket used to cover the person.

Collodions

A gelatin impregnated with medicinal substances for protection and medical effect.

Colocynth *(Citrullus colocynthis)*

The dried fruit is processed to remove the seeds and rind, and the remainder contains a bitter glucoside, which is used as an ingredient in cathartic remedies. It is astringent and tonic, useful in sciatica, colic, and neuralgia. Also called bitter apple, it is a powerful poison which, if administered incorrectly, even in small doses, can cause violent bloody discharges and dangerous inflammation of the bowels. Death has resulted from ingestion of less than 1 teaspoon of the pure powder. The small fruits are sometimes crushed and used to repel moths and small insects from clothing in storage.

Comfrey *(Symphytum officinale)*

There are more than twenty-five species of this herb, populating nearly all parts of the globe, including the United States, where it has been naturalized. It grows in moist locales.

The root and leaves are used, as they are demulcent, expectorant, and astringent, for almost any condition which requires a general cleansing of the entire internal system. The whole plant is made into a tea and consumed more or less freely for complaints such as arthritis, gallstones, stomach disorders, asthma, cancer, anemia, ulcerated kidneys, diarrhea, and female disorders. Externally, it is made into a compress for ruptures, sore breasts, wounds, swellings, bruises, sprains, etc. It is especially well regarded for stemming internal bleeding from wounds or ulcerations.

Compress

A compress consists of a thick piece of cloth wrung out of hot or cold water and applied to some part of the body. A large towel or several thicknesses of cloth should be employed to maintain the desired temperature. Sometimes herbal preparations are added to the water.

Hot compress, or *fomentation,* is used to relieve pain, swelling, and soreness. The cloth should be wrung out from water as hot as can be borne, applied to the body, and covered with a dry towel. This compress should be renewed every twenty minutes and repeated several times.

Cold compress is used to relieve fever, delirium, pain, hemorrhoids, and in cases where stimulation of the cardiac function is desired. Continuous cold application may result in lowered vitality, and placing the feet in warm water during application is sometimes recommended (see *cold pack* in *Cold, therapeutics*).

Alternate hot and cold compresses to the spine are of benefit to the nervous system, the application being changed every five to eight minutes.

Dry heat, considered somewhat less effective than moist heat, is more convenient and does prove satisfactory in many cases. Apply by utilizing electric light bulbs, placed near enough to the body to produce the therapeutic effect. Other means are heating pads, hot-water bottles, hot flannel cloths, and hot salt bags.

Conchgrass (See Triticum)

Confections, Boluses

Pasty masses of herbs triturated while hot (65° C ; 150° F) with sucrose or honey.

Constipating Foods

The following are among the more constipating foods:

white bread	eggs	spicy foods
pastries	rice	white crackers
cornstarch	salted meat	
cheese	pickled meats	

Copper Treatment

European settlers in Rhodesia noticed that African natives who wore copper bracelets and other ornamentation did not develop rheumatic ailments, even though the climate and environmental factors quite likely should have produced them.

Several entrepreneurs have designed and manufactured pure, unalloyed copper devices that are worn as rings, bracelets, and similar items. The treatment is felt to be prophylactic for rheumatism, and is linked in some way with the vibratory radiation of the elemental copper employed.

Coué Autosuggestion

Emile Coué (1857–1926), a French chemist, accidentally gave out a bottle of distilled water in place of a particular medicine. The patient recovered immediately and began recommending the "remedy" to many others. Coué recognized from this experience the major part one's state of mind plays in recovery from all kinds of illness. He founded a free clinic at Nancy at the turn of the twentieth century, and set out upon worldwide lecture tours, delivering a text based upon positive mental thinking and coining a phrase which is still widely repeated today: "Day by day, in every way, I am growing better and better."

Cubeb (*Piper cubeba*)

The unripe fruit of *Cubeb,* cultivated in Java, contains a volatile oil and an organic acid, which accounts for its stimulant, diuretic actions. As a fluidextract and an oil, it is useful for problems connected with the bladder, urethra, and respiratory mucous membranes. Extended use sometimes results in nausea, hemorrhoids, and headache.

Cupping

A method of blood derivation by application of cupping glasses to the surface of the body. A *cupping glass* is a bell-shaped glass capable of holding 3 or 4 ounces, in which air has been rarefied by either flame or suction.

Dry cupping is usually used in inflammatory conditions of the bronchi, lungs, and kidneys. The procedure is as follows: the site selected is moistened with a sponge, and the air inside the cupping device is consumed by applying an alcohol-soaked cotton ball for a few seconds, and then the glass is applied evenly to the skin. The soft tissue within the rim of the cup should swell up and rise into the glass cavity. After about one minute, the glass is removed by tilting, and a surgical blade or *scarifier* is used to make a few minute cuts in the skin, from which blood flows. Two to 3 ounces are usually extracted during one application.

Wet cupping refers to applications in which the skin is cut prior to affixing the cup to the skin.

Sites preferred for cupping are those regions that are fleshy and smooth, such as the nape of the neck, the loins, and the buttocks. All bony parts, and especially the spine itself, should be avoided, as should regions over sensitive organs such as the breasts and at or near any inflamed tissue or skin.

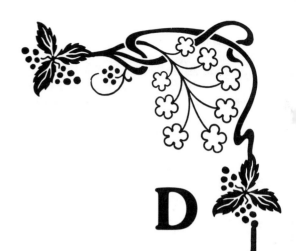

D Vitamin

Vitamin D is one of the fat-soluble vitamins and is a known preventative for rickets, a disease in which less than normal amounts of calcium and phosphate are deposited in the bones. When the vitamin was discovered in 1918, it was realized that more vitamin D is taken through the skin than through the mouth. This makes it unique among the vitamins.

Vitamin D, perhaps the most stable of the known vitamins, is found in small quantities in cod liver oil, egg yolk, and yeast. There are ten compounds which can be converted into vitamin D, and these are labeled D_1, D_2, D_3, and so forth. The two most important of these are D_2 and D_3. Vitamin D_2 comes from a vegetable source, while D_3 comes from an animal source. Often, vitamin D sold in stores will be labeled in this way to identify its source. Both have the same action in the body. Food sources of Vitamin D include fish liver oil (liver of other animals does not contain vitamin D), egg yolk, and mushrooms, which contain the highest concentration of vitamin D except for yeast.

The oils present on the skin are converted into vitamin D by exposure to ultraviolet light, and then absorbed. Once it is inside the body, vitamin D requires the presence of bile to be absorbed from the intestinal tract into the bloodstream. Thus, persons suffering from liver or gall-bladder problems would do better to obtain their D vitamin from a source of irradiation than by tablet or oil.

The recommended dose of vitamin D is 400 units per day, which is sufficient to prevent deficiencies. Up to 10,000 units are prescribed for improving condition of bones and teeth, and 20,000 units to decrease appetite (under a phy-

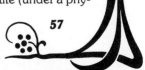

sician's care). While some nutritionists claim that vitamin D can be toxic, the dose would have to be nearly 1,000,000 units per day to produce such an effect. Still, doses in excess of 10,000 units should be supervised by a physician. Vitamin D is also added to fortified milk by direct ultraviolet irradiation. It is also added by feeding cows yeast that has been irradiated with ultraviolet light. It is believed that for children, even a quart of such milk per day does not supply enough vitamin D, and often one of the supplements of oil or yeast is given as well.

Expectant and nursing mothers have extra requirements for vitamin D and are usually advised to take supplements of 1,000 to 2,000 units per day. A considerable amount can be gained while sunbathing in temperate climates.

Decoctions

A 5 percent aqueous solution of vegetable herbs made by boiling the substance (5 teaspoons) for fifteen minutes in a closely covered vessel containing 2 cups of water, allowing to cool, expressing, straining expressed liquid, and adding water through a strainer to make 1 pint. The strength of decoctions of energetic or powerful herbs should be specially directed by a physician or practitioner.

Dentrifices

Finely pulverized tooth powders that are astringent, antiseptic, antacid, non-irritating, nongritty; often sweetened and flavored.

Diaphoretics

Remedies that increase the action of the skin and promote the secretion of sweat.

Simple diaphoretics enter the circulation and are eliminated by the sudoriferous glands, which they stimulate to increase action. Among these are jaborandi, pilocarpus, sulphur, and vegetable salts of ammonium.

Nauseating diaphoretics produce relaxation and the dilation of the superficial capillaries. These include ipecac, opium, warm drinks, vapor baths, Turkish baths, and wet packs.

Refrigerant diaphoretics reduce the circulation at the same time as they act directly on the sweat centers in the spinal cord and medulla. These include jaborandi, pilocarpine, tobacco, cocaine, lobelia, potassium salts, and aconite.

Diathermy

A high-frequency current used to produce heat, especially when it is desirable to reach depths within the body. The diathermy process stimulates cells, glands, and vasomotor nerves, and is recommended in painful or inflammatory conditions such as neuritis, lumbago, sciatica, arthritis, rheumatism, and pneumonia. The current is applied by means of two pads, one usually placed on the part to be treated and one underneath. Other than a sensation of warmth, there is virtually no feeling. Diathermy treatments usually last about ten to twelve minutes. Treatments are applied by registered physicians only. (See *Electrotherapy*.)

Dietetics

Dietetics is the science of the systematic regulation of the diet for hygienic or therapeutic purposes. Proper food is the most important factor in the successful treatment of chronic disease. Nearly all chronic (and most degenerative) diseases are associated in some way with bad diet, and a person cannot expect permanent cure until he or she is educated about correct eating habits.

The human body is composed of sixteen principal elements (see *Body, Chemical Elements in),* and each element must perform a specific duty in the life process. If any are missing, health will be impaired, sooner or later.

The average daily requirement for tissue salts (see *Schuessler Tissue Salts*) is about one-half ounce, and any diet which lacks these amounts is unsuitable. White bread, meat, potatoes, pies, cakes, and most other sweets do not contain mineral salts in proper quantities; what salts are there are driven out and lost in the cooking process.

The meat-potatoes-coffee diet is too rich in acid-forming material; lacking alkaline balance, the acids of fermentation and of the stomach cannot be neutralized. Meat and some cooked foods tend to decay in the alimentary canal, and the gases formed penetrate the intestinal walls and permeate the entire system. The blood in turn becomes congested with waste materials, clogging the capillaries, and a state of autointoxication results. (See *Acid- and Alkali-Producing Foods.*)

The blood is the carrier of the life force, and meat which has decayed in the body destroys or alters the formation of healthy red blood cells. Fruits and vegetables, together with nuts and uncooked cereals, are rich in organic tissue salts, and since these foods do not readily decay or produce toxic elements, they are often employed in greater concentration in diets which aim to restore health to the body.

Natural foods promote all natural functions of the body, keeping the stomach pure and sweet, inducing peristalsis of the intestines, and carrying off toxic matters. Therefore, a natural diet is the first requisite in maintaining and building health.

The six essential food elements are: proteins, carbohydrates, fats, mineral salts, vitamins, and cellulose. Consult these specific headings for further discussion of the food elements.

Digestion

One of the most important functions performed by the body, digestion is both a chemical and a mechanical process. The mechanical process is performed by the muscles, and the chemical process is carried out by the action of the digestive fluids.

The digestive apparatus consists of a tube about 30 feet long, extending from the mouth to the anus, lined with mucous membrane. This tube is called the alimentary canal, or tract, and is composed of the following parts: mouth, esophagus, stomach, and small and large intestines.

Food is taken in through the mouth and moved by action of the tongue, teeth, lips, and gums in an action called mastication. During mastication, saliva, a colorless, alkaline fluid, is secreted by the paratid, submaxillary and sublingual glands. The saliva contains ptyalin, a digestive enzyme, which acts upon the starch in foods, converting it into maltose (this is eventually further converted into simple sugar in the small intestine by the action of pancreatic and intestinal juices). Approximately 2½ pounds of saliva are secreted every 24 hours.

The semisolid food is swallowed from the mouth into the stomach (a process called deglutition). Actually, the food is catapulted along by the action of the pharynx, a small, muscular sac. The soft palate and epiglottis prevent food from entering the nasal passages and windpipe.

In the stomach, the food is changed into a semifluid mass by the action of hydrochloric acid, pepsin, rennin and lipase, substances which are produced by the stomach walls. The food then passes through a sphincterlike valve called the ileocecal valve, which prevents food from being returned from the small intestine to the stomach.

In the small intestine, additional digestive enzymes break the food down further, utilizing three digestive juices: pancreatic juice (see *pancreatin*), intestinal juice, and bile. Bile is not a digestive juice, strictly speaking, but it assists digestion by emulsifying fats and preparing them for the action of other enzymes.

The passage of the end products of digestion from the small intestine into the bloodstream is called absorption. The small intestine is about 25 feet long and has many folds in its lining, which contain nearly 5 million fingerlike projections called villi. These villi present a surface area of approximaely 109 square feet. Each villus contains a central lymph capillary called a lacteal, which is surrounded by a network of blood capillaries. Digested food remains in the small intestine from 5 to 8 hours.

The food now exists in the small intestine as simple sugars, fatty acids, and amino acids each of which is absorbed in a form determined by the action of catalyzing agents. Carbohydrates proceed to the liver, fats are carried via the lymph into the thoracic duct and finally enter the blood, and proteins are absorbed directly into the bloodstream as amino acids.

Fermentative bacteria in the colon, or large intestine, act upon any undigested particles of carbohydrates, producing gases and acids. *Putrefactive* bacteria act upon undigested proteins, producing mainly toxic substances, primarily indole, skatole, and histamine. Indole and skatole are responsible for the offensive odor of feces. Any remaining by-products of a toxic nature are sent to the liver, where they are detoxified and then excreted.

All remaining matter in the colon is acted upon to cause removal of water and then ejected via the anus as feces, composed mainly of skin and seeds of fruits; vegetable fiber; decomposed cellular matter; bile pigments; cholesterol; inorganic salts; and living and dead bacteria, which account for up to one-half of the dry weight of feces.

Diuretics

Agents that increase the flow of urine. Stimulation of the renal epithelium causes increased ejection of the solid and liquid urinary components. Agents that accomplish this include buchu, caffeine, plantain, stillingia, squill, turpentine, juniper, pennyroyal, and uva-ursi.

Diuretics are used to treat dropsy, to cleanse the bloodstream, to dilute the urine, and to stimulate sluggish kidneys.

Pure water is the best dilutant for urine. Irritating diuretics should not be employed in acute inflammation of the kidneys.

Douche Baths

The douche consists of a stream of water propelled with considerable force upon a person, from a height, over distance, or under compression. The size of the stream and its force and temperature are adjusted to the needs of each case.

Douche bathing is recommended for sprains, swellings, and stiff joints externally; and internally for ailments of the nose, ear, eye, throat, stomach, colon, rectum, bladder, vagina, and urethra.

A *percussion* douche is employed in health spas, using a special device to project the water at a pressure between 45 and 60 pounds, gradually decreasing the water temperature from lukewarm to cold. Duration of this douche bath should be short—from one to two minutes.

Dressings

Ointment-like mixtures of powdered herbs heated with fatty base, stirred until beginning to congeal.

Drip Sheet (Sheet Bath)

Often advised in cases of nervous disorders, the drip sheet is applied as follows: the person stands nude in a tub containing warm water to the height of the ankles. A sheet is wrung out of tepid water and cast around the person, covering the entire body. An attendant then virgorously rubs the person with both hands, causing heat of friction to bring blood to the surface of the skin. As the sheet dries from evaporation, new water is applied from a cup or bucket.

The sheet is kept on for about five minutes, and the massage applied throughout the time of treatment. If the person is weak, a stool can be used as support.

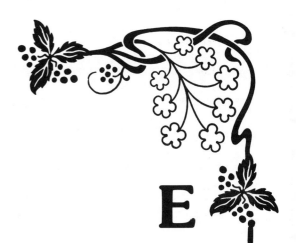

E Vitamin

Vitamin E has gained a reputation for influencing several factors connected with reproduction. One of the most recently discovered vitamins, it has been shown in laboratory tests and practical clinical experience to greatly reduce the risk of spontaneous abortion in women. It also is known that a deficiency of vitamin E in men, over a long period of time destroys the ability of the testes to produce sperm. No amount of vitamin-E therapy can restore the damaged tissue. Beyond these two cases, there is no scientific support for the claims that vitamin E will increase potency, sexual performance, or any other factors connected with sex. But vitamin E is active in other important ways in the body.

Muscles need vitamin E to keep their tone balanced, and thus it can increase the stamina of athletes. In fact, some tests have shown that taking vitamin E increases the heart's endurance by 50 percent, which is a very great increase.

Vitamin E has a dramatic healing effect when applied to the skin; it works by increasing the oxygen supply. Some people squeeze drops from a capsule of the vitamin on wounds, scars, and stretch marks to speed up healing and lessen the effects of scar formation. Cold sores or acid sores in the mouth have responded within twenty-four hours to application of vitamin E.

Vitamin E is fat-soluble but insoluble in water. So for those on fat-restricted diets, it is important that a water-soluble form be used. Even then it must be eaten with *some* fat, to make sure it will be absorbed. Vitamin E is fairly heat stable, which means it can stand most cooking except high heat of outdoor grilling and broiling. It cannot stand light (the ultraviolet rays); for this reason, it is usually sold in dark bottles.

Vitamin E occurs naturally in vegetable oils; good sources are cottonseed oil, corn oil, peanut oil, and wheat germ oil, but not olive oil. Other good food sources of vitamin E are watercress, spinach, lettuce, peanuts, molasses, and legumes. Lesser amounts of the vitamin are found in celery, parsley, and the leaf of turnips. It is also found in meat, butter, eggs and in the fish liver oils.

Like most vitamins, vitamin E is sold in several forms, and considerable confusion exists as to what each is and can do. The scientific name for vitamin E is tocopherol. There are four main tocopherols, the first, or alpha tocopherol, being the one best assimilated by humans. Vitamin E in the natural form is sold as either "alpha tocopherol" alone, or "mixed tocopherols." Naturally, it is more expensive to extract one element of a compound substance, and this is why the pure alpha tocopherol is more expensive than any other form.

There is a further distinction for the alpha tocopherol, which depends upon how the hydrogen is attached to the chemical formula. The best form is known as d-alpha tocopherol. If you use the mixed form of tocopherols, it will have a benefit, but it will also contain some things you do not need and cannot utilize.

Some people confuse wheat germ oil, wheat germ, and vitamin E. Perhaps the richest source of vitamin E is wheat germ oil. Vitamin E is extracted from wheat germ oil. It takes about one cup of wheat germ oil to get the equivalent amount of vitamin E in one 200-unit capsule of d-alpha tocopherol. Naturally, the vitamin-E capsules are more expensive than wheat germ oil. Wheat germ oil is made from the outside covering of the grain of wheat—the germ—which is pressed to extract the oil. Wheat germ flakes are the unprocessed germ, ground up, and are the most economical source of vitamin E.

Wheat germ flakes and wheat germ oil can go rancid, so they should be refrigerated and sealed as tightly as possible. Once they have spoiled, it means that they have been oxidized and taste somewhat "earthy" (as if they need more liquid).

Vitamin E is sold in designations of International Units (IUs), as are vitamins A and D; other vitamins are measured in milligrams. For the average person not involved in heavy physical work or exercise, the dosage of vitamin E is 200 IUs per day. For those who are being treated for heart disease or to rebuild after coronary attack or other illness, physicians have prescribed up to 1600 IUs per day. But such high doses are detrimental if they are begun at that level; it is necessary to build up slowly to that level. The best schedule for taking vitamin E is twice per day with meals. The capsules should be chewed with the food, to ensure that the vitamin has a fat medium to dissolve in. Vitamin E taken alone with a few swallows of water may never dissolve and be wasted. Vitamin E works best when taken with vitamin C, which seems to enhance its action.

The specific physical action of vitamin E is not completely understood, but it is known to affect electron transfers. The body is composed of various elements such as copper, zinc, and hydrogen. Each of these is composed of electrons rotating around a nucleus. The electrons change place at intervals, leaving one element and joining a new one to make new compounds. It is this transfer for which vitamin E is responsible.

Vitamin E is also known to increase the speed and endurance of sperm traveling to fertilize an ovum, to prevent abnormalities in premature infants, and to prevent hair loss. A deficiency of vitamin E is believed to cut down the supply of milk in a nursing mother.

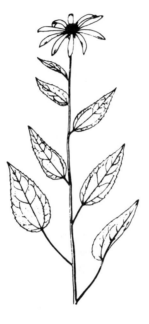

Many of the plains areas of the United States abound with wild-growing echinacea. Herbal applications include use as a natural antitoxin, and treatment for blood poisoning, toxemia, abscesses, and cancer.

Echinacea *(Echinacea angustifolia)*

Known also as purple cornflower, echinacea is native to the plains areas of the United States and is useful in treating all diseases caused by impurity of the blood. Samuel Thomson and nearly all natural physicians have claimed that echinacea is a natural antitoxin. It is used medicinally to treat septic infections, septicemia, blood poisoning, fever, typhoid, abscesses, carbuncles, and cancer. The dosage is 1 teaspoon of ground herb steeped in boiling water for a half-hour. Strain and take 1 tablespoon six times per day. For external application, steep as mentioned and apply or bathe affected part.

Effleurage

A form of massage accomplished by gliding the hands with long, even strokes over the surface of the body. The direction of the strokes, called centripetal stroking, is toward the heart.

Effleurage is done in five ways: with the palms of two hands, with the palm of one hand, with the knuckles, with the ball of thumb, and with the fingertips. The various forms depend upon the part to be treated and the nature of the imbalance. In general massage, for example, there is the opportunity to use the palms of both hands on the long surfaces of the back, legs, arms, and chest. Working on one hand or foot presents the opportunity to use one hand. Knuckle stroking is sometimes employed in foot massage and on the deep muscles of the thigh. The ball of the thumb is employed between muscles, tendons, and the fingers.

The principal benefits of effleurage are that it increases the blood and lymph circulation, soothes the nervous system, and stimulates atrophied conditions of the skin. (See also *Massage*.)

Electric Cabinet

A device for producing radiant heat, the electric cabinet brings on profuse perspiration, thus opening the pores of the skin and assisting in expulsion of toxic matters from the body. The cabinet bath is usually followed by a shower or percussion massage.

Electrolyte Regeneration Program

The "ERP" system, as it is called by its founder, Dr. Robert J. Baumann, D.N. (b. 1940), is a two-fold health approach. Cell nutrition and cell detoxification are involved, and a method of monitoring the body's progress in achieving peak cell efficiency is utilized.

The nutritional portion of the ERP program consists of consumption of foods high in electrical qualities, preferably in embryonic form, such as sprouts, and other foods which have high contents of minerals, vitamins, and enzymes during their early growth periods. The pH of such foods is felt by Dr. Baumann to be such that rapid assimilation into the bloodstream is achieved. Even with proper intake of foods in their ideal form, cell efficiency may be weak if toxic waste and unassimilated metabolic materials are preventing the cell from absorbing the higher-grade nutrients.

Thus a detoxification of the entire alimentary canal is undertaken. Since each person presents a unique health pattern, the ERP program monitors the individual's temperature, pulse, pH, and other visual indicators, which all can be performed by the patient individually with ease. The success of the program has been recorded especially in treatment of persons suffering from degenerative conditions, when used in conjunction with other health approaches.

Electrotherapy

Electricity is a substance made up of rapidly moving electrons traveling at a rate of approximately 180,000 miles per second. An atom, once thought to be the smallest particle of matter, is now known to be composed of many electrons. In one atom of hydrogen, the lightest element known today, there are about 1,800 electrons.

Electrons have a charge, either negative or positive, and it is due to this charge that positive electrons are housed in the nucleus of the atom, while negative electrons can shoot across space or even through other matter such as lead, glass, and wood without touching the electrons of the substance through which they are passing.

The generating of electricity is the separating of the negative electrons in an atom from the positive ones. Whenever a large number of negative electrons leave an atom, it increases the potential of the atom from which they escape, because it is then less "full" of electrons. This action of electron escape is called electrical charge, and the result of it is electrical current. For an electric current to move from one place to another, a conductor is required. The conductor must be well insulated or the current will escape, causing a *short circuit*.

Some terms used in the application of electrical energy include:

> *voltage:* the pressure of electricity, or the amount of power exerted in separating an electron from the atom, measured by the energy needed to push 1 ampere of current against 1 ohm of resistance.
> *ampere:* the measurement unit of the rate of flow, or strength, of electrical current.
> *ohm:* the measurement unit of electrical resistance. Some substances provide less or more resistance to electricity than others. The best conductors of electricity are those offering least resistance, such as silver, copper, and aluminum.
> *watt:* a unit of electrical power, measured as the power produced by an electrical current of 1 ampere passing under the pressure of 1 volt.

Nearly all forms of therapy utilize electricity, directly or indirectly. In natural medicine, the point of view is that all life is a continuous series of electrical impulses, electricity being a vibratory force which, if it is harmonious, results in the balance of life forces. When these forces are unstable, disease occurs. When these vibrations cease, death results. Many chronic and degenerative diseases are remedied by the application of electricity in various forms. Treatment applied at the nerve centers is called indirect treatment; treatment applied directly over an organ is called direct treatment.

The method of application of electrical current for therapeutic purposes is determined by the illness being treated. See *galvanic current, faradic current, static electricity, high frequency current, diathermy, sinusoidal current, ozone, fulguration,* and *Morse Wave Generator.*

Elixir

Sweet, aromatic, hydroalcoholic, medicated liquids; alcoholic strength 20 to 25 percent.

Emesis (See Vomiting)

Emetics

Agents that produce vomiting, emetics are divided into two categories: (1) *local* emetics: act by irritating the end organs of the gastric nerves. These include substances such as alum, mustard, salt, tepid water in quantity, and vegetable bitters, such as quassia or lobelia in strong infusions; (2) *systemic* emetics: general in effect, these act through the medium of the circulation. The principal systemic emetics are ipecac, veratrine, senega, and squill.

Emetics are employed to remove food that is causing irritation or not properly digested, to remove poison that has been ingested, to expel bile from the gall bladder or from the body, and to expel false humours from the channels of the body.

Emmenagogues

Remedies that restore the menstrual function, either directly by stimulating the uterine tissues or indirectly by improving the tone and circulation of the entire system. Direct emmenagogues include ergot, tansy, thyme, wild rue, and digitalis. Indirect emmenagogues are aloe, cod-liver oil, fennel, hot baths, leeching of the genitals, tonics, fresh air, exercise.

A formula to restore menstrual function is as follows:

> 2 tsp. each fennel seed, wild rue, wormwood, and celery seed
>
> 5 figs
>
> 5 tsp. rose hips
>
> 5 tsp. honey

Boil together in 3 cups water for 5 minutes. Take 1-tablespoon doses morning and evening for three days. Stop for three days, then repeat dose for three more days.

Emulsion

Aqueous, milky mixtures of oils, fats, or resins in a minutely subdivided state, suspended by mucilaginous materials; coagulated by acids, metallic salts, or spirituous liquids in large quantities.

Enderlein Therapy

Consists of an isopathic vaccine and sera treatment, and proper diet, based on the work of Dr. Guenther Enderlein, a German zoologist, bacteriologist, and microbiologist who worked in the early twentieth century. He also developed a special blood test which monitors the progress of cancer.

Dr. Enderlein's practical theory was based on the abstract ideas that (1) cells do not represent the final oneness of the living structure, (2) blood is not "sterile," and (3) bacteria undergo an exact, scientifically ascertained development cycle.

The treatment is based on the fact that the lower developmental phases of "endobionts" circulating in the blood can be used as regulators against the higher and virulent pathogenic forms. Endobionts are microscopically and sub-microscopically small organisms, whose development cycle was first described by Dr. Enderlein in 1925. The increased valence of endobionts and their metamorphosis into pathogenic phases parallels the decrease of the quality of the blood and increased intoxication of the entire metabolism.

A full-value and acid nutrition must assist the Enderlein therapy. The injectables include Symbiont-Serum-Enderlein (a symbiont-chondritine), which can also be applied externally, inhaled, or used in tablet form. Literature on the therapy is available only in German.

Enema

A liquid injected by means of a tube into or through the rectum. Warm or tepid water and medicinal herbs are usually added to the liquid, although plain warm water is used as a cleansing wash for the bowel. A fountain syringe is most commonly used.

Enemas are classified according to their action, as follows: *Anthelmintic enemas:* to expel worms, injections are made of salt and plain water or lime water. Also used are infusions of aloe, quassia, or asafetida. *Antispasmodic enemas:* asafetida, lobelia, chamomile, and valerian root are among the effective antispasmodics and carminatives. *Astringent enemas:* ice-cold water will arrest hemorrhage. Enemas of opium are used to check severe diarrhea. Comfrey, lobelia and wild rue are effective enemas in conditions of mucous discharge. *Emollient enemas:* decoctions of starch, linseed, or barley, or of pure linseed oil, will soothe irritable mucous membranes. From 4 to 6 pints of warm water or of milk and water will make an internal fomentation. *Nutritive enemas:* peptonized milk, beef-tea, protein liquid, and eggs beaten together make a good nutritive enema. Four to 6 pints are used at once. Preparations of pancreatin and pepsin facilitate assimilation of the nutritive enema. *Sedative enema:* the enema of *Cannabis sativa* seeds is useful. *Purgative enema:* generally, a 1-pint enema is enough for an adult, 4 to 6 ounces for a child of four years, and 1 ounce for an infant. Soap and water, with or without oil, and glycerin (1–2 ounces) are the commonly employed substances. Large or frequent enemas are not desirable. *Coffee enema:* a therapeutic enema for treatment of detoxification necessitated by chronic or degenerated conditions was developed by Max Gerson, M.D. (see *Gerson Therapy*). The caffeine stimulates peristaltic action and travels up the hemorrhoidal portal vein, and upon reaching the gall bladder, causes it to dump its contents, thereby opening the lines of elimination. One to 2 pints is sufficient.

If frequent enemas are used, they should be followed by a pint of ice cold water to cause the colon to contract back to its original size so that elasticity and peristalsis are not lost.

High enemas, or colonic irrigation, are injections of fluid high into the colon. They are used in cases of extended constipation and as a once or twice a year regimen of keeping the passages of elimination open and clean.

For such enemas, a soft, flexible rubber tube is inserted into the rectum for a distance of about 9 inches. A rubber tube may be coiled at the sigmoid flexure. More often, a metal tube of about 1 inch in diameter and 6 inches in length is inserted into the rectum. This tube is connected to a hose device which injects water into the tube under pressure of from ½ to 2 pounds. After a period, the pressure is turned off, and the contents of the bowels are eliminated via the same tube and passed through a glass tube for inspection. The treatment should be done only by a qualified colonic therapist and lasts about an hour.

Castor-oil and olive-oil enemas are given to soften feces. Six ounces of oil are first warmed and then injected as high as possible in the rectum. A half-hour later, this is followed by an enema of 1 quart of soapy water.

Glycerin is used for purgative enemas (1½ to 2 ounces of glycerin mixed into 1 quart of soap suds). Also for a purgative enema, take 1 ounce salt and 1 ounce of turpentine, mix with 1 pint of warm soap suds. Epsom salts or Rochele salts can be used. Another excellent purgative can be made from 2 to 8 ounces of molasses mixed with 1 pint of soap suds. Molasses can be used alone if it is heated sufficiently to pass easily as a liquid through the enema tube, but not so hot as to cause burning. If molasses is used alone, it should be followed in one-half hour by a soap-suds enema.

To check diarrhea, a starch and laudanum enema is often used. The starch should be prepared the same as for laundry use but made thin enough to pass through the tube. To about 3 ounces of starch, add 30 drops of laudanum. The enema should be injected when it is lukewarm.

Following are the general directions for taking an enema when employing coffee or herbal substances in infusions.

> *Materials:*
> 1. Enema bag with open-pour spout and shutoff valve
> 2. Distilled, nursery, or spring water (the kind sold in glass bottles only)—do not use tap water, as it may contain fluoride, which will not boil out
> 3. Vaseline (for lubricating tip of nozzle)
>
> *Taking the Enema:*
> 1. Hang enema bag not higher than 24 inches above the body entrance.
> 2. Pour one pint of liquid, at body temperature, into enema bag.
> 3. Lubricate nozzle tip with Vaseline.
> 4. Place towel or newspaper around area of buttocks in case of accidental spillage from hose or premature expulsion.
> 5. Lie on right side and gently insert hose tip into anal opening.
> 6. Release hose valve. Liquid will flow into colon. If too much pressure is felt, close valve until pressure stops, then release valve and continue.
> 7. When enema bag is emptied of contents, close valve and remove nozzle tip.
> 8. Retain fluid 10 to 15 minutes (but not longer than 15); then evacuate.

Epsom-Salt Baths

These baths are used with value in the treatment of rheumatism, sciatica, arthritis, tuberculosis, diabetes, toxemia, and so forth. The epsom-salt bath promotes the rapid elimination of uric acid from the blood, thus restoring the blood to its normal condition as an alkaline fluid. To prepare an epsom-salt bath, add about 3 pounds of epsom salts to 12 gallons of water (or a tub half-full of hot water) about 100° F or as hot as can be borne.

The person should remain in the bath for about 20 minutes or until free perspiration occurs. Afterward, cover with blankets or otherwise allow the person to cool down gradually. For therapeutic purposes, the baths are given usually every day for ten days (depending on the condition of the patient), and then every other day until the desired result is achieved.

Ergot *(Claviceps purpurea)*

The spawn (sclerotium) of the fungus *Claviceps purpurea,* growing in the flower and replacing the grain of common rye. The principal action of ergot is to produce artificial anemia and contraction of unstriped muscle fiber. It is used to promote uterine contractions in labor and is very valuable in certain forms of hemorrhage, particularly the postpartum type. One to 2 ounces of the fluidextract are given.

Ergot is also employed in amenorrhea, diarrhea, bleeding hemorrhoids, diabetes, night sweats, vertigo, headache, and tinnitus. It is used locally in gonorrhea, conjunctivitis, and inflammation of the mucous membranes.

Ergot, presently a prescription drug and unavailable through herbal outlets, is listed as an "unsafe" drug by the Food and Drug Administration. Herbalists in Great Britain, Europe, and the Near East are able to make use of ergot without interference.

Eucalyptol

An antiseptic form of camphor prepared from the essential oil derived through distillation of eucalyptus leaves. It is used in malarial fever, bronchitis, and gonorrhea, and locally in nasal application. The dose is 3 to 10 minims, in capsule. Eucalyptol is insoluble in water.

Eucalyptus *(Eucalyptus globulus)*

The leaves (after three year's growth) of *Eucalyptus globulus,* originally native to Australia but raised as a commercial crop in California, contain a volatile oil that yields *eucalyptol* by distillation. In its native state, it is highly antiseptic and antimalarial, and is valuable in treating intermittent fevers. An aromatic bitter, it is also used to promote digestion. Dosage of the fluidextract ranges from 10 minims to 1 ounce.

Expectorants

Remedies that modify the secretion of the bronchopulmonary mucous membrane and promote its expulsion. Primary among the expectorants are: anise, asafetida, black cohosh, bloodroot, cannabis sativa, Irish moss, licorice, lobelia, lungwort, manna, marshmallow, cloves, comfrey, cramp bark, elder flowers, elecampane, fennel, garlic, ginger, ginseng, goldenseal, hops, horehound, hyssop, horseradish, linseed, pleurisy root, pomegranate, sandalwood, sassafrass, senega, snake root, sunflower, stillingia, tragacanth, wahoo, white melilot, white pine, white pond lily, and wild cherry.

Extract

Solid, semisolid, or powdered, made by evaporating medicinal solutions or expressed juices of organic drugs until representing four to five times the strength of the crude substance; these may be aqueous, alcoholic, hydroalcoholic, or acetous.

Eye Washes

Liquid applications for the eyes, usually composed of some astringent salt dissolved in rose water.

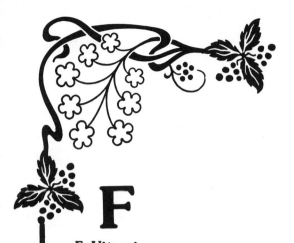

F

F Vitamin

The term vitamin F is somewhat of a misnomer for, rather than being a single substance, it is actually a group of fats known as unsaturated fatty acids (UFAs). Men require about five times as much UFAs as women, but for both sexes it is often difficult to ingest enough of this type of fat.

Unfortunately, frying destroys unsaturated fats, and since the mode of high-heat frying is peculiar to the United States, Great Britain, and the Western world in general, deficiency diseases from lack of UFAs have developed. Cases of psoriasis, ulcers, and some kinds of arteriosclerosis have been reversed by increasing the amount of UFAs in the diet.

The best sources of vitamin F, or UFAs, are wheat germ oil, sunflower seed oil, olive oil, and some fish liver oils. About 2 teaspoons per day of corn oil provide sufficient vitamin F, and unsaturated fatty acids are found in a great many foods in lesser quantities, which makes it rather surprising that deficiencies do occur.

Faradic Current

Faradic current is a rapidly oscillating current of medium voltage and amperage used to cause contraction of enfeebled muscles or to treat paralysis.

One electrode is placed near the origin of the muscle, and the other electrode is placed near the point of insertion of the muscle. Faradic current can be obtained by two or three dry-cell batteries, which makes it applicable for portable use or in remote places without electrical energy. (See also *Sinusoidal Current* and *Electrotherapy*).

Fasting

Fasting is the oldest form of natural correction of physical imbalances. Fasting techniques can range from removal or reduction of one food substance to total abstention from all foods and liquids. Fasts may cover periods from a day or part of a day to more, and there are recorded instances of persons going without food for periods in excess of sixty days.

The idea of fasting is based upon the principle, as stated by the Prophet Muhammad in the comprehensive tradition on medicine, *Tibb-ul-Nabi*, that the stomach is the home of disease.

The food that enters the mouth and is chewed by the jaws undergoes the influence of heat of the mouth (from the body temperature) and the action of enzymes that cause chemical reactions, which again cause heat.

The food is then swallowed directly into the stomach, and the heat of the stomach (hydrochloric acid) "boils" it further, until it is a semifluid mass called chyme—that is, the essence of the digested food. The stomach then sends this essence on to the small intestine, with the addition of bile from the liver. Eventually that part of the food that has become solid sediment is ejected via the bowels, through the rectum. Once these sediments are rejected, the chyme becomes more refined, and the heat of the liver boils the chyme further until it becomes fresh blood. The natural heat of the liver is not quite sufficient to boil the coarser parts of the food, and these become phlegm and bile. The liver then sends these on into the bloodstream and other organs, where further action distributes nutrients to the cells and picks up waste products left from cellular metabolism.

If the process of digestion is off or incomplete at any stage of this continuous "boiling," some organs must work harder than they should to complete the boiling process before it does its own assigned task. Often, other organs of the body must pitch in to assist in other than their primary functions, and thus they become overworked and run-down. Disease, according to this theory, is the end result of such overburdening of the digestive process. Where and how severe a disease is depends upon each person's inherent organ strength and general health.

The logic of fasting is that it stops or greatly reduces the amount of food let into the digestive system, providing time for the body to clear itself of unprocessed foods, superfluities, and harmful pathogens.

A proper definition of fasting, then, would be any reduction of food which engages this mechanism of elimination of superfluous matters. For some, it could be accomplished merely by eliminating meats or sugars from the diet, while for others, it may require total abstinence for some time.

A serious consideration for fasting is that when all food is eliminated for extended periods, the channels of the body become cleared out; so much so that when eating is resumed, if it is not done properly and with great care, these internal channels of the body become clogged with the new amounts of food and great imbalance and illness can result.

Fasting is a purifying process which brings about a rapid elimination of toxic elements from the body. It corrects conditions of disordered nutrition and assimilation, and increases the activity of the eliminative organs, thus helping restore the entire system to health.

The desired result of the fast is to invoke a "healing crisis," which may occur anytime after one or two days or may require two or three months, depending upon the state of health of the person. At this time, the cells have used up all the nutrients which are stored in the body and move from primary digestive work to that of cleansing. This usually is signaled by headache, nausea, dizziness, coated tongue, and similar signs. A healing crisis lasts from a few hours to a day or more and is a sign that the body is passing out toxic matters.

Regardless of the manner or length of fast, it is usually recommended to drink large quantities of water and to keep the lower end of the eliminative organs open by using enemas, either of plain water or other substances which provide nutrients or assist the elimination.

Almost all forms of therapeutic diets are varieties of fasting. The experiences of millions of persons who have used the fast to correct every kind of condition and disease, often after they failed to respond to any other treatment, proves the value of this natural method of cure. Nonetheless, long fasts conducted without proper knowledge or supervision have resulted in severe damage. In many cases, a long fast so weakens the heart and other organs that a recovery is impossible. Safe and scientific fasting, therefore, consists of short, controlled fasts, repeated if necessary at various intervals.

Fats

Food is divided into three main categories; proteins, carbohydrates, and fats. A typical fat molecule has much more carbon and hydrogen than either of the other two types and needs more time and energy to be oxidized. When oxidation does take place, heat is released, and this is what is measured as "calories" of food intake.

Fat insulates against heat, allowing for comfort in hot weather. Fat is necessary for sexual maturity, pregnancy, and lactation. Vitamins A, D, E, and K must have fat present in order to be assimilated, and fat by its physical presence holds several of the internal organs in place, such as the liver.

Fatty acids also are believed to protect the body from the effects of X-ray radiation, whether from the environment or diagnostic machines. Some signs of fat deficiency are retarded growth in children, scaly skin, kidney lesions, and eczema.

The assimilation of fat occurs within the small intestine. Up to 50 percent of the fat consumed is converted into fatty acids, and the rest eliminated in the feces. Vegetarians, who generally consume much fewer fats from meats, generally have a greater incidence of gallstones because the gall bladder stores fats to process bile salts. If these fats are not "digested," they turn into hardened deposits or stones.

Obesity, or "fatness," is a condition in which the accumulation of fat reserves is so great that the function of organs is interfered with. Obesity can be caused by a decrease in exercise, making less need for fats, or because the body is not breaking down the fats, which increases fatty deposits.

Feces

All the substances that are formed by food in the process of digestion and mixed with various secretions of the body are eventually emitted from the body via the rectum. Various chemical substances, microorganisms, and worms may also be present in the feces.

Fennel (*Foeniculum vulgare*)

Fennel was well known to the ancients, who used it to strengthen sight. In medieval times, it was used as a preventative for witchcraft and evil influences. While the root was used in former times, today only the seeds are used medicinally. The odor of fennel is sweet and fragrant, and its properties are best released in hot water. A formula for improving and balancing the digestion is made by taking 1 teaspoon of fennel, half-crushed, 1 teaspoon of powdered ginger, and enough honey to make a thick paste. Use ½ teaspoon of the mixture in a cup of hot tea after meals. Fennel is also employed as a carminative, a cholagogue, an expectorant, and a galactagogue.

Fermentation

Fermentation is a general name for the processes of decomposition which affect any composite humid substance. During this process, a chain reaction is set forth which affects the carbon compounds of the substance. The *ferments* produced by these chemical changes are of two types: *enzymes,* or *organic* ferments, which have no definite structure and are not living, such as diastase, ptyalin, and pepsin; and *organized* ferments, which are microscopic, living organisms, such as plant molds, bacteria, and other types of the lowest form of plants, the protophytes.

Fevers

The first sign of many illnesses is fever. Fevers occur when the natural heat of the body is insufficient to complete the process of "boiling" in each stage of digestion (see also *Fasting*).

When the body has received what it needs to sustain itself, it eliminates the unassimilated excess, along with any natural excess, in the form of sweat, tears, mucous, and so forth. But often the body cannot expel this unassimilated excess arising from overeating or eating foods containing chemicals which the body cannot digest. This excess remains in the veins, the liver, and the stomach and increases with time. Any composite humid substance that is not boiled and processed undergoes putrefaction. Such putrefaction may occur in any limb or organ anyplace in the body, causing a disease to develop in that part. Anything in a process of putrefaction generates heat, and this heat is what, in the human body, is called fever.

Rise of temperature is the most prominent feature of all fevers and can be determined by the use of a thermometer placed in the mouth, axilla, rectum, or vagina. The mouth is usually preferred. The normal termperature for each of these sites is:

axilla or groin	98.4° F
mouth	98.6° F
rectum or vagina	99.5° F

The terms to indicate degrees of feverishness are:

feverishness	99° to 100° F
slight fever	100° to 101° F
moderate fever	102° to 103° F
high fever	104° to 105° F
intense fever	in excess of 105° F
hyperpyrexia	106° F and above

A person undergoing a healing crisis with fever should rest in bed in a quiet room that is well ventilated with adequate warmth. A doctor or skilled medical person should monitor the progress of the healing crisis so that the fever does not get out of hand.

Nutritious foods should be given, preferably of a liquid nature, in small quantities. The eliminative tract must be kept open, with enemas if necessary, and diuretics and laxatives as well. Pure water should be given in quantity.

Sometimes the temperature rises so rapidly and to such a degree that it is desirable to lower it or bring it under control. This can be accomplished by hydrotherapy, using cold packs, cold baths, sponge baths, and herbal drugs, which must be selected by a natural physician.

Generally speaking, addition of cold foods to the diet can help lower the temperature. Cucumber, yogurt, tomatoes, lemons, oranges, and green teas are all helpful. It must be remembered, however, that fever is the body's own healing way of processing out congestive, superfluous matters. It does not make sense to suppress a fever entirely, for it will merely drive the excesses deeper into the body, making a more difficult healing crisis inevitable in the future.

Finsen Light

The ultraviolet rays of the light spectrum are called finsen light. They have been used in the treatment of *lupus vulgaris*, a rare type of skin tuberculosis. The rays of this light are weak and do not penetrate very far into the skin. (See also *Heliotherapy*.)

Flaxseed (See *Linseed*)

Fluidextract

Solutions of organic drugs evaporated until 1 cubic centimeter represents the activity of 1 gram of crude drug.

Fluoride

Fluoride is a chemical substance usually extracted from aluminum wastes. Many of the most prominent physicians and scientists have condemned its addition to water supplies, yet the practice continues as a "preventative" of dental cavities in children and adults. The National Health Federation has used its staff of scientists and researchers to attempt to block further use of this chemical treatment of water. While some studies have shown that fluoride does lessen incidence of cavities, it has also been shown to produce cancer in laboratory tests on animals. It is a subject of great controversy.

Fluorine

A trace mineral present in bones and teeth, it occurs naturally in garlic and watercress. Since such a small amount is required by the body, normal consumption of vegetables provides adequate amounts.

Fomentations

Flannels wrung out of hot water and applied with or without medication.

Food, Classification

The following chart presents the basic food principles and the types of foods in which they are found:

Classification of Food Principles

1. Proteins

Principle	*Source*
myosin	flesh of animals
vitellin, albumin	yolk of egg, white of egg
fibrin, globulin	blood contained in meat
caseinogen	milk, cheese
gliadin and glutinin	grain of wheat and other cereals
vegetable albumin	soft, growing vegetables
legumin	peas, beans, lentils, etc.

2. Fats

animal fats and oils	adipose tissue of animals; seeds
stearin, olein	grains, nuts, fruits, and other
palmitin, fatty acids	vegetable tissues

3. Carbohydrates

saccharose, or cane sugar	sugar cane
dextrose or glucose	fruits
levulose, or fruit sugar	fruits
lactose, or milk sugar	milk
maltose	malt, malt foods
starch	cereals, tuberous roots, leguminous plants
glycogen	liver, muscles

4. Inorganic Principles. Water; sodium and potassium chlorides; sodium calcium, magnesium, and potassium phosphates; calcium carbonate; and iron.

5. Vegetable Acids. Malic, citric, tartaric, and other acids, found principally in fruits.

6. Accessory Foods. Tea, coffee, alcohol, cocoa, etc.

Food, Rules for Combining

Not all foods agree with all people all of the time. It is impossible to construct hard and fast rules for food consumption or combination, because in specific cases, such rules could be contradicted or even harmful. What is required is a sensible study of each person's dietary needs and health goals, and with competent guidance and education, one should arrive at the best diet for each individual. Nearly all recommendations for food intake are for what is required by the "normal" or "healthy" body, which is a rare specimen. The following rules for combining foods are generally true, but are subject to alteration depending upon various diet factors and health goals.

1. Acid foods are best eaten alone and not with foods of the starch category such as potatoes, rice, and bread. Acids may be eaten with fatty foods, which help reduce the irritations in the stomach that consumption of fruits may cause.
2. Acids should not be eaten with protein foods, since proteins tend to cause fruit acids to coagulate.
3. Foods which have approximately the same digestive times should be eaten at each meal. (See *Foods, Digestion times* in Appendix A).
4. Fats should not be consumed at meals with starches or proteins, because fats coat the lining of the stomach and hinder digestion of these substances.
5. Foods eaten at one meal should be restricted to two or three of the same category. Vary categories at each meal.

Food, Suitable Diet

Innumerable efforts have been made to estimate the proper amount of protein, starch, and fats for the "normal" person. No rule has been established, but the amounts below are accepted today as proper ranges:

protein	50 to 60 grams
fat	100 to 125 grams
starch	250 to 550 grams

Foxglove *(Digitalis Purpurea)*

Made of dried leaves of the *Digitalis purpurea,* foxglove contains no alkaloid, but five glycosides—digitalin, digitoxin, digitalein, digitonin and digitin—are derived from it. Four of them are heart stimulants. Digitonin is a heart depressant.

Digitalis stimulates the heart and regulates its rhythm, slows the pulse, and acts as a diuretic. It is used medically for weakness of the heart, syncope, collapse, dilation of the heart, and poisoning by cardiac stimulants. The medicinal form of digitalis is extracted only from the leaves of the plant.

Herbal pharmacopoeias list other uses, such as for treatment of fresh wounds, dropsy, internal hemorrhage, delirium tremens, epilepsy, and mania.

Foxglove should be administered only with medical supervision, as continued use leads to an accumulation of the drug in the system and to hypertrophy of the heart muscle.

Friction

Friction is a type of heat generated by rubbing two objects against one another. In natural therapeutics, it refers to the production of heat for the purpose of massage, to bring blood and oxygen to an area, to reduce the effects of cold, and so forth.

Friction may be produced by the thumb, tips of the fingers, or palms of the hands, and is best generated by circular motion toward the center of the joints. The purpose of friction is to limber the joints, tendons, muscles, and skin, to break up deposits of toxins and to reduce swelling and nerve inflammation.

Fructose

Fructose, also known as grape sugar or levulose, is a white, crystalline substance. Honey is about 39 percent fructose.

Fruit Diet

The chief value of fruits is due to the sugars, mineral salts, vitamins, and acids they contain. Since fruits contain acids which are converted into carbonates in the blood, they keep the blood more alkaline than it would be otherwise. Fruits also have value as laxatives and for their beneficial effect on the digestive organs. Cleansing fasts of grapes, oranges, apples, peaches, grapefruits, and other fruits are often employed for a few days to reduce the toxic matters in the system (see *Grape Diet*). A simple, cleansing fruit fast consists of eating three meals per day comprised of two oranges and one apple per meal. Variations may be used. Eight glasses of water per day are recommended for the duration of the fast. If it is desired to extend the diet for a longer period, milk may be added as a protein source.

Fruits, Acid and Subacid

Fresh, uncooked fruits supply digestive chemicals and natural sugar and also phosphorous compounds for the brain, nerves, spinal cord, and bone marrow.

The acid fruits (those below 4.0 pH) are: lemon, pineapple, tangerine, orange, grapefruit, rhubarb, lime, cranberry, grape, tomato, apple, strawberry.

The subacid fruits (those above 4.0 pH) are: apricot, blackberry, cactus fruit, cherimoya, cherry, elderberry, gooseberry, grape, guava, huckleberry, jujube, mango, nectarine, papaya, papaw, peach, pear, persimmon, plum, quince, raspberry, sapodilla, and sapote.

Fulguration

Fulguration, or electrocoagulation, is a process which destroys cells and coagulates tissues. A similar process, *dessication,* dehydrates tissues, causing them to shrink up into a dry mass. A special electrode is used for fulguration, consisting of a needle and a probe with which to point it; these are connected to an electrical generator. The sparks are discharged from the needle point directly into the tissues with extreme rapidity. (See *Electrotherapy.*)

Warts, moles, tumors, and other tissue growths, and tattoos have been successfully treated by this electrical process. Usually one or two treatments is sufficient to destroy small growths such as warts.

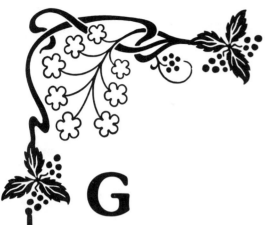

G

Galactagogues

Herbs that increase the flow of milk. Among those plants which accomplish this function are aniseed, blessed thistle, buckwheat (as a poultice), carrots, fennel, jaborandi (small), red raspberry, and vervain.

Gall Bladder

The gall bladder is a pear-shaped bag about 4 inches long and 1 inch wide at its greatest diameter, holding from 8 to 12 fluid drams. It is lined with a mucous coating and is situated in a fissure on the undersurface of the liver. The *cystic duct,* about 1½ inches long, joins with the hepatic duct at an acute angle to form the common bile duct through which bile manufactured in the liver passes to be stored in the gall bladder.

Galvanic Current

One of the most widely used electric currents, galvanic current is continuous and can be obtained from a machine using wet or dry batteries or directly from commercial current. The most favorable results are obtained from low voltage (40 to 80 volts) and low to medium amperage.

To employ galvanic current, two contact points are used, thus forming a current of electricity which passes through the body. The current is taken in through the positive pole and passes out via the negative pole. The properties associated with each pole follow.

Positive Pole	*Negative Pole*
attracts oxygen	attracts hydrogen
accumulates acids	accumulates alkalis
contracts arterioles	dilates arterioles

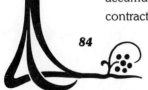

stops bleeding	stimulates
sedates	softens tissues
hardens tissue	alkaline caustic
acid caustic	increases bleeding
hard and unyielding	soft and pliable

The galvanic current stimulates the life force and increases the functional activity of the parts through which it passes. The effects of the treatment last longer than the time of application of the current, usually for several days. Galvanic current excels in producing contraction of the muscles, thus strengthening weak muscles.

Often a pad is attached to each line of current, and the negative and positive poles are placed to produce the most stimulation of the specific organ needing treatment. There are also many electrodes made for inserting into various orifices of the body, such as the rectum, vagina, urethra, and so forth.

Medical doctors, naturopaths, and chiropractors are the physicians who most often employ galvanic current in their treatments. (See also *Electrotherapy*.)

Gamboge

A resinous gum from *Garcinia hanburyi,* a tree native to southern Asia. Due to the presence of an acid, it is a severe hydragogue cathartic, extremely diuretic. Dosage of the gum is 2 to 5 grains, and it is used as a component in cathartic pills.

Gauzes, Carbasi

Gause muslin, free from sizing, saturated with a medicated solution of a definite strength, and then spread horizontally to dry.

Gentian

The root of yellow gentian is a bitter tonic and is used in cases of dyspepsia, malaria, jaundice, and as a vehicle for cod-liver oil. The dose of the fluidextract is 1 to 5 grains; of the tincture, ½ to 2 grains. The dose when used in an infusion is from ½ to 1 teaspoon in hot, sweetened water.

Gerson Therapy

This therapy is described in detail in the book *A Cancer Therapy—Results of Fifty Cases* by Max Gerson, M.D.

Before Dr. Gerson came to the United States, his reputation in Germany was highly esteemed by such honored men as the late Dr. Albert Schweitzer. In fact, he saved the life of Dr. Schweitzer's wife. Dr. Schweitzer, himself a medical doctor, said of Gerson, "I see in him one of the most eminent medical geniuses in the history of medicine. . . . Many of his basic ideas have been adapted without having his name connected with them."

Dr. Gerson first came to the attention of the medical profession and the public in 1929, when he developed an effective dietary treatment for tuberculosis of the skin (lupus), which had been considered incurable. The treatment tries to reinstate the natural, normal, biological balance of the body and is based on complete detoxification, or internal cleansing, of the body, based on the functioning of the liver.

The liver is the most vital organ in recovery from any disease. The sick liver does not function well enough to purify the blood and to reactivate the oxidizing enzymes. Dr. Gerson blamed a high sodium(salt)-to-potassium ratio in the liver for contributing greatly to the inception of cancer. This undesirable ratio affects the metabolism of fats and proteins, causing poisonous substances to develop.

A special diet, as salt-free as possible, and potassium medication are used to restore proper liver function. In some cases, to help reactivate the liver, castor oil is given by mouth and by enema during the first two weeks of treatment in addition to the all-important coffee enemas which, in advanced cases, are given every four hours, day and night, for the first two to three weeks. The absorbed caffeine from the coffee enema travels through the portal veins directly to the liver and there opens the bile ducts and stimulates the bile flow, which contains the toxins and poisons, and eliminates them. The Gerson method takes patients off all drug sedation, since poisons must be eliminated from the body.

When the liver and digestive track are reactivated and brought into order, the local cancer symptoms disappear because the accumulated poisons which caused the cancer are eliminated. The treatment also acts to restore the necessary enzymes.

The Gerson therapy is generally undertaken for a period of one and one half to two years to assure effective treatment.

Dr. Gerson's method is a medical treatment which must be applied by a physician after thorough examination and correctly adapted to each patient's individual needs. It requires supervision and regular follow-ups by the attending doctor. Neither the dietary regime nor the medication is effective alone—the combination is essential for success. Gerson was said to have had a 40 percent cure rate.

Ginger, Wild *(Asarum canadense)*

Also called Canada snake root, Indian Finger, and Vermont snake root, ginger appears as many different species and changes in appearance depending on the area in which it grows. It is native to the United States, growing from Maine to Michigan. The more valued species for medicinal purposes are imported from Africa, India, Pakistan, and China.

The root is fleshy and round, deep green on top and light green below. It is a very good medicinal article, having a warming and agreeable effect upon the stomach. It is a powerful stimulant and is not volatile, as are many other hot herbs. It is used as a substitute for cayenne when the latter is not available.

The best method is to obtain fresh roots and grind or pound them to a fine powder. The dose must be adjusted to the circumstances; if it is given to raise the internal heat in order to cause perspiration, it must be repeated in teaspoon-size doses until it has the desired effect. Ginger makes an excellent poultice when mixed with pounded cracker or slippery elm bark.

Keeping a piece of the root in the mouth, chewing it like tobacco, and swallowing the juice is excellent for a cough. This should also be done by anyone exposed to contagious diseases, as it will guard the stomach against taking the disease.

Ginger may be taken as a tea beverage in hot, sweetened water.

Ginseng *(Panax quinquefolium)*

Panax quinquefolium has many common names. Research from all over the world indicates that many millions of people agree that ginseng is one of the most useful herbs known to humans.

It is native to China, eastern Asia, and other parts of the world, but that which grows in North America from eastern Canada to Maine and Minnesota and southward into the Carolinas is considered by some to be the best in the world.

As a wild plant, it grows up to 20 inches high, with three large leaflets and a yellowish cluster of flowers which are produced in midsummer, then followed by bright red berries.

The root is the desired part. It is thick and, on older, larger plants, somewhat resembles the human body in shape. It usually takes six or more years for the root to reach a size that is marketable.

The roots are gathered best in autumn and then dried for use. Ginseng was known and used by many people mentioned in the Bible, and in recent history, the American Indians used ginseng as a medicine and exported it to England in the seventeenth century.

Taken as a tea, ginseng stimulates the production of pepsin and thus is an excellent digestive aid. It has the ability to stimulate malfunctioning endocrine glands and is a powerful antispasmodic in diseases such as asthma. The

Chinese have created a legendary place for ginseng through their use of the root for a wide array of conditions, including neuralgia, indigestion, weak heart, spinal and nervousiaffection, poor circulation to the brain, as a potent tonic to regenerate and rebuild the sexual glands, and as a cholagogue and an expectorant.

Ginseng is known to give off organic radioactive rays which stimulate vital processes in living cells. It is used for treating children as well as adults, but in adjusted doses.

To make ginseng tea, use 3 ounces of seven- to eight-year-old ginseng in a powder, add 1 ounce of honey and 60 ounces of wintergreen, and blend them together. Use one teaspoonful to one cup of boiling water, and boil it lightly for ten minutes. Drink as hot as possible.

There are several dozen ginseng products on the market today, with proponents swearing by their own favorite varieties. Considerable literature is available, but one of the best texts is *The Complete Book of Ginseng,* by Richard Heffern, published in 1976 by Celestial Arts, Millbrae, California.

Girdle Pack

The girdle or abdominal pack is one of the most effective compresses. It has a beneficial effect on the stomach, spleen, liver and solar plexus, relieving chronic congestion of these parts. The girdle pack is constructed by taking a piece of thick cloth long enough to reach entirely around the body. The cloth is wrung out from cold water and placed around the abdomen. Over this wet pack, a dry piece of woolen cloth or Turkish towel is wrapped and fastened securely. The pack is then left in place for several hours or overnight.

Gluten

Gluten resembles albumin and is identical with it chemically. It is found in large amounts in the seed of cereals, in the form of cells surrounding the starchy fecula of the seed.

Gluten bread is a kind of nonstarch bread used by diabetics. It is made as follows: Take 1 quart of fresh cow's or goat's milk, or equal parts of milk and water; 1 heaping teaspoonful of pure butter; 1 /5 of a cake of compressed yeast beaten with a little water; and 2 eggs well beaten. Stir in enough gluten flour (about 3 cups) until a soft dough is formed. Knead as you would in making regular bread. Put in pans and let rise. Bake in hot oven until brown.

Glycerin

A viscous, syrupy, colorless substance derived from certain fats, such as those of palm oil, by decomposing them under superheated steam. Glycerin is highly antiseptic, abstracts water from the tissues with which it comes into contact, and, unless it is very pure, is often irritating to the skin. When it is taken internally, it acts as a laxative, and thus glycerin suppositories are often employed to relieve chronic constipation. It is also used to soften crusted matter in the external ear and as a preservative in syrups and other herbal mixtures.

Glycerites

Solutions of an herb in glycerin for external use.

Glyoxylide

A nontoxic, injectable medicine discovered by the late William F. Koch, M.D., Ph.D., in 1919 and part of the Koch treatment for cancer and many other diseases, including allergies and infections.

Glyoxylide, a patented trade name, is a catalyst which restores proper oxidation in body cells and converts toxins to antitoxins in a chain reaction where dehydrogenation (removal of a hydrogen atom) initiates oxidation in the cell and destroys the pathogens integrated with the cell.

The theory is that insufficient oxidation due to the accumulation of toxins in the body is a necessary factor in cancer and nearly every other disease. It was Koch's belief that the cancer germ or virus is originally harmless but becomes virulent when poisoned by the toxins in the system.

According to Dr. Koch, cancer cells have lost both the capacity to conduct oxidation and also the mechanisms that use the energy produced by oxidation. Since oxidation does not occur in the affected cells, the energy is transferred to other cells, forcing increased cell division; thus the cancer becomes parasitic upon the rest of the body.

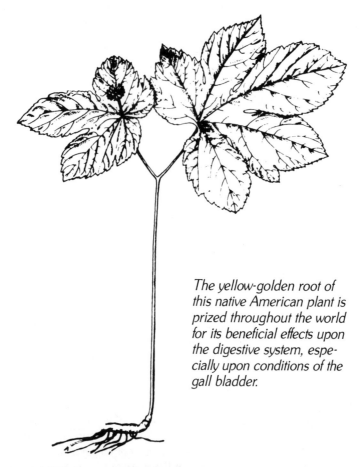

The yellow-golden root of this native American plant is prized throughout the world for its beneficial effects upon the digestive system, especially upon conditions of the gall bladder.

Goldenseal *(Hydrastis canadensis)*

Goldenseal is native to North America, growing perennially in the Eastern parts. The rough yellow root, which is the part used medicinally, contains several alkaloids. The fresh root is quite juicy, and this juice was used by the Indians as a dye.

Goldenseal is an excellent bitter to correct weak digestion that causes distress. One teaspoon of the powdered root in hot water gives almost immediate relief. It is also a superior corrector of the bile and is a specific for hemorrhages of the pelvic tissue. Externally, it is employed as a lotion in treating skin diseases and eye afflictions, and for general cleansing.

The dose of the powder is from 10 to 30 grains; of the tincture, 1 to 2 fluid teaspoons. The roots can be prepared by placing 1 teaspoon of the powdered root in 1 pint of boiling water. Let stand until cold, and drink 1 to 2 tablespoons three to six times per day.

Granulation

Caused by the formation of dextrose crystals in liquid honey. By applying a low heat for ten minutes, these crystals usually can be eliminated.

Granules

Very small sugar-coated pills, ¼ to ½grams; parvules are still smaller and usually contain poisonous alkaloids or chemicals. *Dragee* (dra-sha) is the name given in France to the ordinary sugar-coated pill.

Grape Diet (Grape Cure)

The grape diet gained currency by being employed in European health resorts for treatment of a variety of chronic disorders, from constipation to cancer. The diet is arranged in the following manner:

Beginning the first day, 2 pounds of grapes are eaten, increasing 1 pound daily until the maximum of 12 pounds per day is reached. No other foods are allowed.

Another method is eating 2 or 3 pounds of grapes three times per day, consuming 6 to 9 pounds per day total.

The grapes should be black or red, fresh and ripe, and of course thoroughly washed. This is a most excellent diet for constipation, autointoxication, and other chronic disorders, but best carried out under the supervision of a doctor or other health practitioner.

Grape Sugar (See *Fructose*)

Guelphe Fast

The Guelphe fast restricts, or eliminates, all forms of solid and semisolid foods and in their place allows consumption of nutrient substances in the form of juices and liquids. Fruit juices, vegetable juices, and broths are allowed, but there should be no pieces of vegetable in the broth.

Diabetics are sometimes advised to take up this fast, as a predomination of one kind of juice or substance can be useful, such as carrot juice, lettuce juice, herbal teas, and so on.

The fast can be employed for up to two days without interruption, but twenty-four hours is usually the limit, and it is effective within that time.

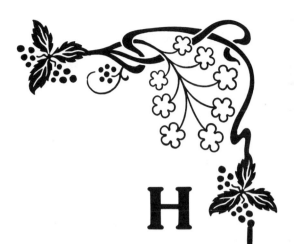

Hallucination

The highest degree of subjective sensation, dependent only upon the stimulation of the sensory cortical centers. There is perception of nonexistent objects or impressions, which are creations of the imagination. Hallucinations can be classified as hypochondriacal, motor, pseudosensorial, unilateral, visual, auditory, gustatory, tactile, and so on. Hallucinations may be caused by ingestion of LSD, marijuana or *Cannabis sativa,* peyote, and other plant and mineral substances. They may also be present without ingestion of any substances, such as during high fevers or extreme emotional states.

The Healing Crisis

Every imbalance that is corrected by the body's own healing mechanism has four steps: addiction, growth, crisis, and decline.

The stage of *addiction* occurs when the body is exposed to the actions or substances that are ultimately the cause of the disease. During the time of *growth,* the substances are accumulated—or for germs, grow without the body's defense mechanisms being brought into action. In *crisis,* the body acts to repel the cause of the disease, whatever its nature. The crisis may happen at any stage of the disease and be quite sudden, or it may appear mildly from time to time even during the growth period.

The crisis occurs at different periods due to the nature of the substances causing the disease and the means being used to correct it. The body is never idle but sometimes must assume a status of standby, just waiting for the substance to be refined enough to be thrown off.

The disease can be considered an enemy and physical health a king guarding his territory. The day of crisis can be compared to the day of battle. On fighting day, the king has complete control over how he will use his fighting forces to repel the enemy: suddenly attacking, mounting all the troops for a big attack, or splitting them into fighting factions.

As on a real fighting day, both sides provide the weapons of the battle, and the terrible sounds of cries of battle can be heard. The person feels fear and anxiety, hears voices, and rough and abrupt movements shake his body.

On the day of the healing crisis, the person should never be stimulated, for if the stimulant works in the same way—in agreement—with the natural healing mechanism, it will weaken the natural disease-repelling force. If the stimulation works against the natural repulsive faculties, the body's nerves and inner systems will become confused and nature is prevented from complete action: the substance is not taken out fully and the disease is not completely eradicated. Thus, on the day of crisis, avoid herbs that provoke diarrhea or vomiting or other stimulation and avoid as much as possible feeding the person.

Crisis, in terms of substance repulsed, has five modes: vomiting, diarrhea, nosebleeding, urination, and perspiration. Crisis by urine or perspiration is incomplete because a thin substance is thrown out and a thick one remains. Crisis by vomiting, nosebleeding, or diarrhea is complete.

If the crisis is to happen during the day, the signs appear the night before, or vice versa. Each crisis is preceded by its own signs. For example, the signs of crisis by vomiting are asthma, change in breath rhythm, bitter taste in mouth, cardiac pain, stomach convulsions, lowered pulse, and trembling of the lower lip. The signs of diarrhea are intestinal pain, heaviness of body, stomach gas, backache, colored feces, and grumbling intestines. The signs of crisis by nosebleeding are dull sense of hearing, ringing in ears, tears, itching nose, and beating of veins in head. Signs of urine crisis are heaviness of urinary bladder, thickness and excess of urine, bright color of urine on fourth day of illness, and with the full crisis occurring on the seventh day. The signs for each type of crisis usually occur alone, but may combine in various ways.

One should pay attention to the process of crisis, to see if the substances are expelled with force. If not, the elimination is incomplete and a doctor must be consulted to complete the repulsion of the substances.

The correction of disease occurs from the top of the body downward and from the inside outward. Thus, the first sign of a crisis often is headache, lastly diarrhea. Furthermore, in the process of the correction of the body, the order of signs is acute, subacute (between acute and chronic), chronic, and degenerative. The first signs in the acute stage are swelling, heat, redness, and pain. If the body can repel the substance or correct the inharmony at this stage, it will. If not, the disease will be driven further into the body and become chronic. This stage may last weeks or years, depending on many factors. When the chronic stage is not corrected, organ damage occurs and the signs of degenerative disease are present.

The stage of *decline* arrives as the crisis passes and harmony is restored.

It is easy to see that the best time to correct any condition is at the first sign of imbalance. It will take less time and less effort and will be healed more quickly. In correcting during the chronic and degenerative stages, the disease must be traced back through each of the stages it went through in arriving at its advanced condition. This is why, when people are able to recover health through natural medicine, the last signs of healing are often the *same ones* that occurred when the disease first began. Those trained in natural therapeutics know how to recognize these signs and effectively manage the healing crisis.

Heart

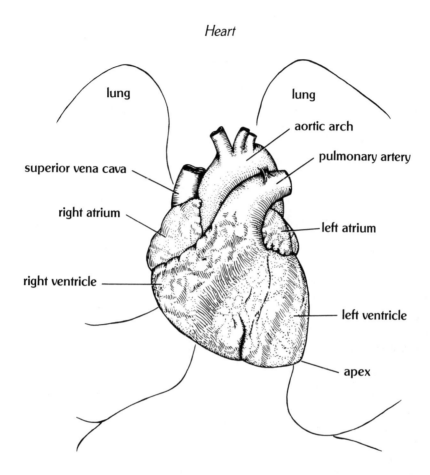

Heart

The heart is a hollow muscular organ shaped somewhat like a cone, located in the chest on the left side between the lungs. In adults, it measures about 5 inches by 3½inches and weighs 8 to 12 ounces.

There are four cavities in the heart—an auricle and ventricle on each side. The right and left arteries proceed from the aorta or main artery, and the veins accompany the arteries and terminate in the right auricle. The nerves are derived from the cardiac plexuses, which are formed partly from the cranial nerves and partly from the sympathetic nerves.

According to humoral medical theory of the East, the heart serves the additional function of being the seat of manufacture and storehouse of the breath, a concept rejected by Western scientific theory.

Heliotherapy

The treatment by direct rays of the sun is called heliotherapy. As an empirical treatment, it is as old as history, but as a scientific method, it has only been brought into use by Western doctors in the past several decades.

The sun has a temperature of approximately 8,000° C or 14,000° F, and is the most powerful source of heat and light in nature, being vital to the life process itself.

Subjected to a prism, sunlight breaks down into the colors of orange, yellow, green, blue, indigo, violet and ultraviolet. Red and orange are heat rays; green and yellow are light rays; and violet and ultraviolet are chemical rays.

The longest visible rays are the red rays, but the invisible heat waves of the infra-red rays are even longer. Beyond these are the hertzian waves, named after Dr. Heinrich Rudolf Hertz, who discovered them in 1877. The invention of the wireless telegraph was possible only because of the discovery of these invisible waves. There are also other shorter rays, such as the radium gammas and Roentgen rays.

The principal therapeutic value of sunlight is derived from the ultraviolet rays and the chemical or actinic rays. It has been demonstrated that these rays will penetrate into the cells of an organism and increase the metabolism of that part or body. This action simultaneously modifies the effects of oxidation, bacteria, tissue growth, and pain. The rays of the sun have been used to stimulate or improve many conditions, including poor digestion, blood problems, lymphatic congestion, and skin diseases. Sunbaths taken inside lose some of their effectiveness, as the ultraviolet rays cannot penetrate through glass.

In treatment of diseases by sunbaths, the person is usually exposed nude to the sun, allowing the rays to reach the whole body. In some circumstances, the whole body cannot be exposed, and thus disrobing of at least the torso area is advised, as this part of the body contains the greatest number of important organs. Beds and chairs can be moved in front of an open window to take advantage of the sun if a person is bedridden.

The first sunbath in a treatment should not last more than ten minutes, to avoid burning sensitive skin. The time can be increased gradually until the person is able to sit in the sun up to one or two hours per day. Headaches, skin redness, slight fever, or blistering are signs that exposure has been excessive.

Hellebore *(Veratrum viride)*

American hellebore contains jervine, veratrine, and other alkaloids. It is a powerful depressant of the heart and is paralytic to the spinal cord, and is thus used as a circulatory sedative in acute inflammations such as pneumonia, pleurisy, and peritonitis. It is contraindicated in conditions of depression or if vomiting is feared. Hellebore is poisonous. The preparations of the plant in common use are the fluidextract (dosage 1–4 drops), the tincture (dosage 10–30 drops), and as a tea, either singly or combined with other herbs.

Hemlock *(Conium maculatum)*

Hemlock belongs to the same family of plants as parsley, fennel, parsnip, and carrot, but it is a potent poison. Its primary use in ancient times was as a poison administered to criminals, and it was the fatal poison which Socrates was condemned to drink.

Hemlock has been used as an antispasmodic and a sedative, but due to the possible fatal side effects, it is definitely not recommended for general herbal use.

Henry VIII

The British king formally protected herbalists by a proclamation in 1542 that has come to be known as the Herbalist's Charter. At that time, physicians were split into two categories: those who employed only herbs, and those who employed any substance—including chemicals—which they felt had a place in treatment, even though the side effects may have been more dangerous than the original disease. While the Herbalist's Charter had some effect in protecting early American colonialists, the first herbal doctor in America, Samuel Thomson, was persecuted for utilizing only herbs in his treatments.

Herbalism

Treatment by herbs is the oldest known form of therapy, with reference to applying herbs found as far back as the Chinese text *Pen Tsao* (3,000 B.C.), which contains about a thousand remedies using plant substances.

The origins of herbal medicine are lost in the mists of antiquity and certainly predate all existing records. Early humans, who had the intelligence to construct tools and to paint on the walls of their cave dwellings, could not have failed to observe the correlation between items of diet and the functions of the body.

They would note that an attack of diarrhea was corrected by certain astringent fruits and leaves; that the discomfort following overindulgence in food was relieved by the ingestion of the mints; that mucilaginous roots and leaves soothed irritating coughs; and that certain leaves applied to abraded skin eased pain and accelerated healing. Through this empirical process, a body of sound herbal knowledge was compiled and transmitted from generation to generation.

So important did this information become to the community that it was committed to a caste of priest-physicians. Medicine, one of the earliest professions, became associated with magic, religion, and astrology. The art of healing appears in this form in the earliest records we possess.

The medical papyrus discovered by Georg Moritz Ebers in Thebes dates from 1550 B.C., and the Chinese medical treatise, *The Yellow Emperor's Classic of Internal Medicine,* written some thousand years earlier, contains discussions of the therapeutic uses of plants mixed with ideas of astrology and metaphysics.

During the Eightieth Olympiad (around 460 B.C.), the Hippocratic school separated herbal medicine from the occult and related it again to a careful observation of the patient. Hippocrates, in his work *On Purgatives,* formulated the principle that treatment and dosage should be decided in accordance with the individual patient's requirements and idiosyncrasies.

Accurate description and definition of medicinal plants was the special contribution of Theophrastus in the third century B.C.; he became the father of botany as well as of pharmacognosy. His history of plants includes descriptions of five hundred species that are used medicinally.

The art of medicine and the use of botanical remedies declined under the Romans in the early centuries of the Common Era, as shown by the mere 185 plants in the standard herbarium of Lucius Apuleius. But the Anglo-Saxons have left records of at least five hundred medicinal plants and their uses. From the Norman Conquest until the time of the early printed herbals, little is known of herbal medicine apart from the work of Bartholomew the Englishman, written about 1260.

The Dutch herbal of Rembert Dodoens (1517–1585), translated into English by Henry Lyte in 1578, formed the basis for the 1597 herbal of John Gerarde and for the largest herbal printed in English, which was compiled in 1636 by John Parkinson and which contained descriptions of the medicinal use of some 3800 plants.

Herbals published in following centuries consisted mainly of the rewriting, without acknowledgment, of earlier works. Some authors, like the quasiherbalist Nicholas Culpeper, attempted to take herbal medicine back into the obscure world of astrology and the occult. Authors such as Culpeper are repudiated by contemporary herbal practitioners; their ideas are not consistent with those generally accepted by herbalists and give the false impression that herbal medicine is atavistic and archaic. Nothing could be further from the truth.

Since 1965, work has proceeded with the preparation of definitive, authentic monographs on medicinal plants used at the present time in the British Isles. Part I of this work, the *British Herbal Pharmacopoeia,* has now been published by the British Herbal Medicine Association. The description of each plant is prepared by pharmacognosists from the pharmacy schools of the University of London, and the therapeutic section is derived from the recorded observations of senior herbal practitioners who are members of the National Institute of

Medical Herbalists. The pharmacopoeial committee, established by the British Herbal Medicine Association, includes scientists, botanists, pharmacists, and medical herbalists, with medical practitioners as advisory members.

During the early 19th century, Samuel Thomson (1769–1843) caused the spread of herbal medicine into the major portion of the population of the United States. He wrote a classic work, *Guide to Health; or Botanic Family Physician* (Boston: J. Q. Adams, 1835) which set forth his principles of applying herbs to regain health ("heat is life and cold, death"), and contained many formulas which are still—and even more widely—in use in the United States today.

Thomson was persecuted by the orthodoxy of his time, and spent several extended periods in jail. Ultimately his detractors, members of the medical establishment, had him arrested on charges of murder, after one of his patients died in the course of Thomson's attempting to treat a terminal illness. The case was heard during a special sitting of the New York State Supreme Court, and Thomson was acquitted even before being allowed to present his defense.

Most of the activities of herbalists in the United States have been influenced by the Thomsonian System, which was rooted in the practice of humoral treatment originated by Hippocrates.

During the eighteenth century, the discovery and isolation of volatile oils, organic acids, and alkaloids from plants laid the foundations of phytochemistry and of the pharmacological approach to herbal medicine. Since that time, the number of herbal remedies in the official pharmacopoeias of the West has progressively diminished, but over the last quarter-century, research interest in botanical *materia medica* has increased notably.

The plant kingdom has been explored by widespread screening programs such as that carried out by Norman Farnsworth and his colleagues in Illinois. The number of plant species has been estimated at 800,000, the greater proportion of which has not yet been examined phytochemically. A recent report has stated that more than one thousand species of plants not previously investigated have yielded alkaloids, many of which are biodynamic. The possibilities for the discovery of further potent therapeutic agents from plant sources are immense, and this field invites active research.

Clues about which plants are likely to be suitable for investigation are often derived from the reputed therapeutic action of herbs in folklore. The Cancer Chemotherapy National Service Center of the United States has examined the legends on herbarium labels and documents dating back to 2838 B.C. for indications of plants used by people for the treatment of malignant and nonmalignant tumors. R. E. Schultes (1972) states that many thousands of plants are reputed to demonstrate anticancer activity, and as a result of the investigation, the active principles of more than fifty of these plants have been isolated and their structures elucidated.

Herbal medicine, as practiced today, is multidisciplinary and requires knowledge of the normal and pathological states, of plant *materia medica* and of pharmacology. The practice is characterized by a number of principles which may be regarded as corollary to the contention that sickness is often best treated by the use of naturally occurring plant remedies. The herbal practitioner places emphasis on some of these widely accepted principles to guide him in his approach to therapy.

While admitting the undoubted value of specialization, medical herbalists are, at heart, general practitioners. They are unhappy about the degree of specialization that is characteristic of much medicine today. They regard each patient as an individual, and after careful, time-consuming diagnosis, they prescribe herbal remedies for that person's needs. In any practice, for two patients to receive the same prescription would be entirely fortuitous, however similar their symptoms.

Herbal practitioners are free from restrictions of standard formulations or dosage forms but exercise their skill and experience in preparing "tailor-made" prescriptions for their patients. On subsequent visits, progress is assessed by monitoring the appropriate parameters, and any necessary adjustment is made to the balance of the prescription.

Some herbal practitioners prescribe a mixture of dried, comminuted or powdered herbs, but most prefer herbal remedies in the form of liquid preparations as extracts or tinctures. A liquid extract is prepared by percolation, extraction, and concentration at a low temperature and under reduced pressure to minimize oxidative or hydroxylative changes in the plant constituents and to avoid loss of volatile and thermolabile substances. The final product is a one-to-one preparation, that is, 1 milliliter of the liquid extract contains constituents from 1 gram of the dried plant. Tinctures also are prepared and adjusted to pharmacopoeial standards. The concentration of a tincture is frequently standardized at one-fifth of the liquid extract.

By administering remedies in liquid form, fine adjustments to the prescription are facilitated as treatment proceeds. This is necessary because no two persons—with the possible exception of monozygotic twins—share the same internal environment and microsomal enzyme processes. The same dose administered to a group of patients may result in up to a fortyfold variation in plasma concentration—or even more in some recorded instances.

Although the main processes of absorption, protein binding, metabolism, storage, and excretion are understood, our knowledge of how the human body operates is far from complete, and other factors that determine the availability of drugs to the body remain unidentified. The *holistic* concept of the patient, which results in specific treatment for the clinical syndrome and individual treatment to suit the patient's personality, is of great importance.

One objection that has been raised against herbal remedies is based upon the variability of constituents and their concentration in different specimens of a medicinal plant. Therapeutic potency is thus variable within certain limits. A considerable amount of research is in progress to define more exact standards for herbal remedies than the current determination of ash value, volatile-oil content, or general assays that are required by the pharmacopoeias. Chromatographic techniques are being applied to this problem in many parts of the world, from the United States to China, and the resulting standards will enable qualitative and quantitative assays to be performed on each batch of herbal material, crude or processed. Many indeterminates will then be removed, but the complete solution to the standardization of herbal remedies will not be found until clinical and pharmacological evidence has indicated each of the therapeutically active constituents. Constituents readily amenable to chromatographic assay are not necessarily a useful index of the therapeutic potency.

In an era characterized by widespread publicity, one may wonder why so little is heard of herbal practitioners and their work. Part of the reason is that they have no desire to proclaim their therapy from the housetops but are content rather to quietly pursue their call to heal. Their reward, in common with that of all true physicians, is to receive the gratitude of their patients.

When the media present herbalists, they are usually portrayed as parodies based on folklore or native practices; not surprisingly, the erroneous assumption is made that medical herbalism is a vestigial remnant of a murky past. However, the roots of herbal medicine are securely planted in recorded observations of current practice and of past generations, and impart stability to the profession in a period of unprecedented change.

For too long, herbal practice has been restricted by ignorance, misconception, and even prejudice. Before this century is out, we may expect research to release from the plant cell effective remedies for the killer diseases which now defy treatment. The plant kingdom, which is the source of the food we eat and the oxygen we breath, will thus provide for humankind the medicine of the future.

It should be noted that the foregoing discussion centers mainly on the development of herbal medicine according to the European/British historical model. Long before the rise of codified herbal practice in Europe and Great Britain, the Islamic cultures of the Middle East and throughout the Indian subcontinent had a fully developed system of herbal pharmacopoeia. In fact, the *British Formulary* was, until the eighteenth century, based upon the famous work of Avicenna, the *Qanun-ul-fi-Tibb*. (See also *Arab Medicine, Avicenna, Tibb-i Unaani*).

High-Frequency Current

A very rapid oscillatory current of high voltage and low amperage, the high-frequency current is so fast that the sensory nerves are unable to respond to it, thus making it one of the safest and least painful of electrical treatments.

By passing many millions of minute electrical charges through the body, each cell, muscle, nerve, and organ is stimulated without discomfort.

The two best-known forms of high-frequency current are the Telsa and

D'Arsonval, and nearly all high-frequency machines are variations of these two. The Telsa Coil discharges a high voltage, low amperage current, while the D'Arsonval is of low voltage and high amperage current. The electrodes are of various forms, for application to specific parts of the body. Some practitioners form their own from tin or other conductive substances.

The effect of these high-frequency currents is to increase the volume of blood and lymph flowing to parts of the body, which results in oxygen and nutritive stimulation. It also acts to remove waste and superfluous products from the area of disease. (See also *Electrotherapy*.)

Hippocrates based his system upon the concept of physis, *meaning the organism in its unity. According to Hippocrates, disease occurs when the digestion* (pepsia) *is being carried on with great difficulty* (dyspepsia).

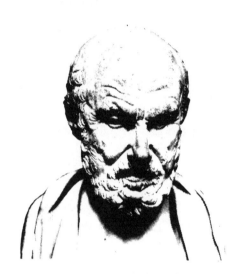

Hippocrates

Hippocrates, often called the Father of Medicine, was born about 460 B.C. (d. 357 B.C.) on the Greek island of Cos, to a long line of priest-physicians. He traveled widely throughout Greece and is known to have founded a medical college at Cos.

Hippocrates' medical theories, which are still partly accepted, were based on the concept of *physis,* meaning the organism in its unity. Unlike other, earlier philosophers who tended to separate people from their environment, Hippocrates insisted that there was some life force greater than the organism, and that was Life itself. In the constant interaction of the organism with its environment, the organism grows at the expense of the environment, taking from the environment what is necessary for life and rejecting what is unnecessary. In this interaction, according to Hippocrates, disease occurred when there was severe difficulty in the digestion (*pepsia*) of the environment by the organism, or *dyspepsia*.

Hippocrates left no truly codified science, and his reputation today rests chiefly upon the Hippocratic Oath.

Hippocratic Oath

The Hippocratic Oath is recognized as having genuinely originated with Hippocrates, but the exact time and circumstances are not known. Here is the full oath:

> I swear by Apollo the Healer and by Aesculapius, by Hygeia and Panacea, and by all gods and goddesses, making them my witnesses, that I will fulfill according to my power and judgment this oath and this covenant. I will look on him who taught me this art as I do my own parents, and will share with him my livelihood. If he be in need, I will give him money. I will hold his offspring as my own brethren, and will teach them this art, if they wish to learn it, without fee or written bond. I will give them instruction by precept and by lecture and by every other mode to my sons, to the sons of him who taught me, and to those pupils who have taken the covenant and sworn the physicians' oath, and to none other besides. According to my power and judgment, I will prescribe regimen in order to benefit the sick, and do them no injury or wrong. I will neither give on demand any deadly drug, nor prompt any such course, nor, similarly, will I give a destructive pessary to woman. In holiness and righteousness I will pass my life and practice my art. Into whatever houses I enter, my entrance shall be for the benefit of the sick, and shall be void of all intentional injustice or wrongdoing, especially of carnal knowledge of woman or man, bond or free. And whatsoever, either in my practice or apart from it in daily life, I see or hear which should not be spoken of outside, thereon will I keep silence, judging such silence sacred. If then I fulfill this oath and do not violate it, may I enjoy my life and art and be held in honor among all men for ever; but if I transgress and prove false to my oath, then may the contrary befall me.

Homeopathy

Homeopathy is a safe, scientific, logical system of medicine founded by Dr. Samuel Hahnemann in 1796. It is based on the axiom, *similia similibus curantur,* ("like cures like"), also called the Law of Similars.

In homeopathy, no drug or substance is given which can produce a toxic effect, but rather minute doses of remedies are given to stimulate the defense mechanism of the body to heal itself.

The homeopathic *materia medica* contains more than two thousand different remedies, with descriptions of even the smallest variations in symptoms. Homeopathic remedies are prescribed in various potencies, with the higher potencies being actually further dilutions of the smaller doses. A 1X potency, for example, is obtained by taking one part of the substance, and diluting it with nine parts of water, alcohol, or sugar (honey can be used). A 2X potency would be obtained by taking one part of this 1X remedy and further diluting one part of that with ten more units of base. The potencies must be made according to homeopathic pharmacological procedure, which can produce potencies in very high ranges, such as 200X, 1000X, and even higher.

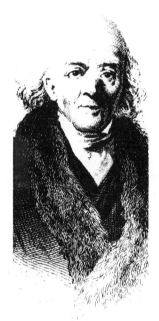

Samuel Christian Hahnemann (1755-1843), founder of homeopathy.

In the 1920s in the United States, all homeopathic physicians were medical doctors who received advanced medical training in homeopathy, which was a subspecialty of medicine. The orthodox medical doctors, however, had severe differences with the homeopaths, and as a result of persecution, most homeopaths went out of practice or underground. Today there are only a few medical doctors who practice homeopathy and a few lay practitioners. Some effort is being made to revive the science. In 1978, for example, there was a bill before the Arizona State Legislature to legalize homeopathy, and in California, lay practitioners are allowed to administer remedies as long as certain warnings are made known to the patient. In Europe, many respectable homeopaths practice, including the official physician to the present Queen of England.

Honey

The nectar obtained from flowers by worker bees and some other insects, honey is a viscous fluid collected by bees for use as their food.

Aristotle called honey "the dew distilled from the stars and rainbow," and honey is widely mentioned in the Bible and Koran as a healer and remedy. The nutritive elements of honey are absorbed into the bloodstream extremely fast—within ten minutes—which makes it one of the most useful applications for skin diseases and afflictions.

The chemical analysis of honey is as follows:

water	20.5 (per cent)
ash	0.2
protein	0.25
ideatroix	36.8
levulose	32.35
cane sugar	1.30
substances not fully classified	8.60

The nutrient minerals in honey are sodium, 16.9 milligrams per 100 grams; calcium, 0.51; and phosphorous, 32.

An interesting text presenting the many uses of and historical information about honey is *Honey as Healer,* edited by Lionel Stebbing (Sussex, England: Emerson Press, 1975).

Hops *(Humulas lupulus)*

Humulus lupulus, or hops, contain inpulin as its most important principle. It is a chologogue, an expectorant, a bitter stomachic, is slightly hypnotic, and also causes a slight increase in cardiac action. It is most widely used as a mild nervine, either as a tea or by itself or in conjunction with herbs such as valerian, peppermint, and chamomile. A poultice of hops is a favorite to relieve painful conditions and inflammations. An infusion of tea is often used, or a fluid-extract, in doses of 5 to 15 minims.

Horehound *(Marribum vulgare)*

Horehound is the most common of the plants in the mint family, and while it is native to Europe, it has found its way to wild growth in the temperate zones of North America, growing in practically all parts of the country in dry, sandy fields and wastegrounds and by roadsides. The entire plant has fine, white, downy hairs, and small white flowers appear as blooms.

Horehound has mainly been used to treat coughs and bronchial afflictions, asthma, colds, and all complaints of the lungs. An infusion of the leaves is utilized for all the foregoing conditions, and a tablespoon of syrup of horehound will usually loosen tough phlegm and relieve the signs of a hoarse cold. Horehound is also popular made into a candy, and "cough drops" with horehound as an ingredient have been popular for nearly a century. Large doses are laxative and have been used to expel various types of intestinal worms. For children, the dose is 1 teaspoon in 1 pint of water to make a tea. Add honey and drink freely for coughs and colds.

Horseradish *(Armoracia rusticana)*

Once known as *Cochlearia armoracia,* both the root and leaves of horseradish have been used in natural medicine since the Middle Ages. While the root has been used in the United States primarily for culinary purposes, its extreme hot nature makes it suitable for medicinal action especially as an expectorant. Since horseradish is very volatile, the warming qualities, so evident when eating, are almost entirely diminished before reaching the stomach. The roots may be given, however, to promote the appetite, and the leaves are sometimes applied as a poultice to remove external pain, but should be used with caution as blisters are sometimes raised. An infusion of sliced horseradish root mixed with milk can be used as a cosmetic for clear, smooth skin.

Hot-Air Treatment

The physiological effects of hot air are: temporary increase in circulation, respiration, and fever; moderate local anesthesia; loss of weight due to loss of water from skin and lungs; and decrease in output of nitrogenous matter.

Hot-air treatment is employed as a treatment for lumbago, acute sprains, acute rheumatism, and stiff and contracted joints. For acute, painful conditions, hot-air baths may be given every other day, or every day, if necessary. Chronic cases should be treated less frequently.

For sprains, the hot-air treatment is usually sufficient to relieve all pain. The hot-air treatment of joints renders them flexible and softens up adhesions. Manipulation of the joints of the spine is more easily accomplished right after hot-air treatment. Body temperature, respiration, and pulse are all slightly elevated during and just after hot-air treatment. (See also *Bier's Hyperemic Treatment; Sweat Baths.*)

Hot Packs

A hot-blanket bath, or hot pack, is administered by placing a rubber sheet and one or two woolen blankets on the bed. A heavy woolen blanket is wrung out from water at 110° F, spread on the dry blanket and the person wrapped up like a mummy. The dry blankets and rubber sheet are then placed around the person, who is kept inside this pack for one-half to two hours.

A wet hot pack is made by using a single sheet wrung out from hot water and spread upon a dry blanket, in which the person is wrapped similarly to the above procedure. After an hour, the pack is removed and the person rubbed lightly for a few minutes with cold cloths (65° F).

Hoxsey Herb Treatment

This treatment was made famous by Harry M. Hoxsey, M.D. Estimates of the number of cancer patients cured by the Hoxsey method range from 25,000 to 75,000. In fact, a U.S. congressman discouraged Dr. Hoxsey from carrying out a plan to have 25,000 of his cured patients picket the White House.

The major Hoxsey formulas have been changed several times; the exact ingredients and dosages vary depending on the patient's general condition, the location of the cancer, and the extent of previous treatment.

These formulas can generally be compounded by a good druggist on a doctor's prescription. The herbal medicines could also be obtained from a good herbalist.

Humoral Medicine (See *Tibb-i Unaani*)

Hydrastis (See *Goldenseal*)

Hydrochloric Acid

A liquid composed of about 32 percent hydrochloric acid gas (HCl) and 68 percent water; it is used as a caustic and to stimulate the salivary and alkaline digestive secretions. When given in small doses before meals, it relieves acidity of the stomach and has reportedly been effective in preventing dysentery. Diluted hydrochloric acid (10 percent) can be used, but a more convenient form is betaine hydrochloride, obtained from beet tops.

Hydrochloric acid is an ingredient of the gastric acid secreted by the gastric glands. The hydrochloric acid is produced in the stomach by the parietal cells. The amount of hydrochloric acid present in gastric juice varies from 0.2 to 0.5 percent by volume.

Hydrochloric Acid (HCl) Therapy

This treatment was developed by Burr Ferguson, M.D., and Walter B. Guy, M.D., and described in the book *Three Years of HCl Therapy,* originally published in 1935 by W. Roy Huntman, Philadelphia, Pennsylvania.

It is maintained that there are five underlying factors which allow the formation of neoplastic growths or cancers:

1. A deficiency of potassium in tissues.
2. Potassium deficiency causes loss of function, particularly in posterior spinal nerves, which normally control reproduction of cell life.
3. Hypochlorhydria is the chief cause of potassium deficiency.
4. Hypochlorhydria, likewise, causes alkalosis of tissues.
5. When a group of cells becomes isolated from nerve control, such cells become a parasitic entity. Iron is precipitated into lymph channels, blocking the affected areas from the lymph circulation and nerve control of cell life, and these blocked lymph areas become a fruitful field for microorganisms to infect these occluded tissues.

Dr. Ferguson believes that potassium deficiency, which is quite common, may be due to a hypochlorhydria brought on by worry, grief and so on, producing a deficiency of hydrochloric acid and thus giving rise to lactic acid replacement and maldigestion of food and impaired absorption of mineral salts.

By supplying potassium in a hydrochloric acid solution, a rapid improvement appears not only in cancer victims, but also in people with lymph stasis of heart tissues seen in angina pectoris, myocardiac cases, congestion and failure of pancreatic cells as seen in diabetes, and anemias of the blood.

Hydromel

Also known as mead, hydromel is a honey beverage, often dispensed by Galen, suitable for invalids and persons of weak constitution. Made of equal parts of honey and water, it soothes the mouth and stomach and stems feverish conditions.

Hydrotherapy

The restorative powers of water are due to the fact that it equalizes circulation, increases muscular tone and nerve force, improves digestion and nutrition, and increases the action of the perspiratory glands, thus eliminating dead or damaged cells and toxic matters. Treatment is by baths; the nature of the bath determines the specific effect. For therapeutic purposes, baths are classified according to the temperature of the water, as follows:

Temperature	Duration	Effect
very cold, 32–43° F	a few seconds, only under supervision	tonic
cold, 40–60° F	30 sec.–2 min.	tonic, shocks nervous system
cool, 60–72° F	30 sec.–3 min.	invigorating; improves circulation
tepid, 80–90° F	5–7 min.	cleansing; lowers fevers, cools inflammations
neutral, 92–95° F	1–2 hours	refreshes; aids burns
warm, 90–100° F	15–30 min.	equalizes circulation; reduces pain, softens skin
hot, 100–105° F	8–10 min.	relieves pain; aids neuritis and skin eruptions
very hot, 105° F & over	few seconds– few minutes	relaxes; reduces muscle spasms, dilates blood vessels, raises blood pressure

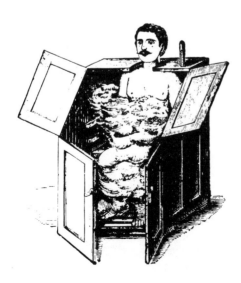

One variant of hydrotherapy, the steam bath, is conducted in a cabinet. The steam is introduced into the box via a hose which is attached under the seat. Beneficial effects of hydrotherapy include increased muscular tone, improved digestion, and elimination of dead cells and toxic matters.

Care should be exercised not to overdo hydrotherapy treatments and to make certain that the body can endure the temperature which is employed. Local applications can be made in place of or in preference to total immersion. Water is seldom applied over 120° F, and complete immersion in water above these temperatures is very dangerous. The human body can tolerate vapor up to 140° F and dry air above 300° F, but these temperatures are not recommended.

Warm baths are sedative if they are prolonged; cold baths are stimulating if short and depressing if extended; hot baths are depressing temporarily. Alternating applications of hot and cold baths will produce strong stimulation. If they are used in alternation, the cold application should be only about one-third the duration of the hot application.

It must be remembered that the oily secretions of the skin serve a purpose, and if they are removed by too frequent bathing, a disordered condition of the skin can result.

Hypnosis

An artificially induced state of mind or mental attitude in which the powers of volition and action are altered, and during which it is sometimes possible to force a person to commit acts which would not readily be accepted at other times of normal consciousness.

Hypnosis is employed to restore certain normal functions (such as in cases of psychosomatic paralysis), to remove false impressions upon the subconscious (phobias), to restore self-control, to correct evil thoughts and bad habits, and to relieve painful states. Hypnotism has been used with benefit to produce anesthesia.

There are many conflicting opinions as to what hypnosis is and how it is produced. Usually there must be a feeling of genuine trust between the therapist and the one being hypnotised. In spite of strange performances by lay hypnotists on entertainment stages around the world, hypnotism has gained a respectable place in modern medical treatment, with sometimes remarkable results achieved in diagnosis of disease with the patient's cooperation while under hypnotic trance.

Hypotonic Therapy

A method for treating cancer and many other ailments was discovered by John T. Stephens in 1957. The method consists of regular intramuscular injections of pure, sterile, distilled water, although other nontoxic solutions of hypotonic concentration (i.e., of osmolarity less than that of body fluids, which is equivalent to the osmolarity of a 0.9 percent saline solution) can be used.

The mechanism involved is a nonspecific reaction, triggered by injection, releasing enzymes, hormones, and cell chemicals which have nontoxic, beneficial, normalizing effects throughout the body. The diluted injected fluid passes through the cell walls of tissue at the injection site and, in accordance with physical laws governing osmosis, increases the fluid volume inside the cells until they burst, releasing their contents into the circulatory system. The tissue heals rapidly, leaving no mark, and no permanent damage is incurred when the fluid is injected as described.

Varying benefits have been noted in cancer, leukemia, cataracts, arthritis, senility, other degenerative type diseases, and virus infections. Improvement in chronic conditions can be expected within one to several months; viruses respond within days, with possible accompanying fever.

Hyssop *(Hyssopus officinalis)*

Hyssop is of the mint family and has been used as a cleansing herb and purifying tonic to the body since Biblical times. It is valuable as a treatment for colds and sore throats, as a blood regulator, and for asthma, among other conditions. An infusion as a tea can be taken in cup doses several times a day. Hyssop is applied externally as a poultice to relieve bruises and is used commercially in the production of wine, food, and cosmetics.

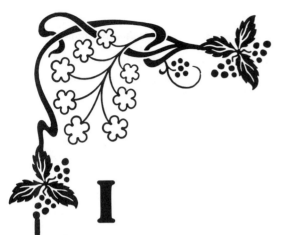

I

Ice

Ice is a refrigerant, an analgesic, a hemostatic, a sedative, an antisecretant, and an antiphlogistic. It is applied in several ways: as cracked ice, iced compresses, and suppositories, or by means of an ice bag, ice cap, or ice poultice. It is employed in cases of angina, hemorrhages, various inflammations of the eye, chronic vomiting, dysentery, and similar afflictions.

Indian Healing

The term *medicine* has meant something quite different to American Indians than it does to American white society. The Indian art of healing was based on ceremonial ritual. Indians knew that the process of healing is intimately tied to the spiritual state and station of the patient. While the Indian healing rituals may seem inexplicable to us today, we still have various ritualistic modes in treatment, namely, the sending of get-well cards and flowers to the bedside of the sick. Even the way of undressing for and being touched by physicians is highly ritualistic.

According to Alma Hutchens, when the first Anglo explorers landed at Plymouth Colony, they found the Indians of New England had names for only sixty-six diseases. In 1924, Herbert W. Youngken, a pharmaceutical historian, synthesized a list which presented a total of 450 plant remedies used by the Indians. Modern medicine, however, combats approximately twenty thousand diseases with tens of thousands of drugs.

The basis of Indian medicine is strikingly similar to that developed in the East by Hippocrates, Galen, and Avicenna; namely, that heat, sun, hydrotherapy, and similar natural modes were employed along with herbal remedies. Likewise, the training of an Indian healer was by preceptorship, and a long period of apprenticeship was required before a healer was allowed to work on the sick. The notion of the body being made up of the four elements—earth, water, air, and fire—was, of course, central to the Indian concept of healing.

Unfortunately, orthodox medical people have not thought well of Indian medicine until the previous decade. References to the Indian medicine man are usually derogatory.

Today, however, traditional Indian medicine men and women and other healers are participating in an important resurgence in the popularity of natural healing, and several authoritative texts have appeared which have given some added credibility to the rich traditions of Indian healing. An excellent text on this subject is *American Indian Medicine* by Virgil J. Vogel (New York: Ballantine, 1973).

Indian Hemp (See *Cannabis Sativa*)

Indican

Indican, a toxin, is derived from indol, a product formed in the intestines by the putrefaction of protein foods. In a normal body, only trace amounts of indican are present in urine. Larger amounts of indican are found when the intestinal contents undergo rapid decomposition, as during intestinal indigestion, disorders of the liver, and peritonitis. It is also found in excess in urine in cases of abscess of the lungs, appendicitis, and empyema.

Infant Development

There are no hard-and-fast rules which can be said to apply for every infant. Most parents want their children to be "above-average." The following guides for growth and development are averages, and reaching a particular height and weight and the ability or lack of ability to perform certain tasks at certain ages have no particular significance. If a parent is concerned about reflexes or other abilities of an infant, a physician or practitioner should be consulted.

Generally speaking, then, the following are only general guidlines regarding infant development:

A child should be able to hold up its head by the fourth month, to sit up by the seventh month, to walk by the twelfth to eighteenth month. The "soft spot" on the rear of the skull should harden and close at the second month, and the one on the front part of the skull should solidify at the eighteenth to twentieth month.

Weight and Size (Average)—The height of girls is about the same as boys; the weight of girls about one pound less.

At birth	7½ lbs.	20 inches
At 6 months	16 lbs.	25 inches
At 1 year	20 lbs.	29 inches
At 2 years	26 lbs.	32 inches

Growth can be reduced due to poor nutrition, impure air, and certain diseases such as scrofula. Also, other disorders can greatly accelerate growth, such as some forms of endocrine imbalance.

Infant Feeding

Children fed at the breast should have milk at regular intervals, approximately according to the following chart:

Age	Intervals	Number of Feedings in 24 hours	Number of Night Feedings
From birth to 4 weeks	2 hours	10	1
4–6 weeks	2 hours	9	1
6–8 weeks	2½ hours	8	1
2–4 months	2½ hours	7	0
4–10 months	3 hours	6	0

The breasts should be kept scrupulously clean and washed after each feeding especially. The baby can be allowed to nurse for about fifteen minutes but should not remain at the breast more than twenty minutes at a time. Nor should a baby be allowed to fall asleep while nursing. Usually the best results are obtained by alternating the breasts at each feeding time. Breast feeding should be discontinued when the child reaches age two.

Infusions

A 5 percent aqueous solution of herbs made by adding to the substance (5 teaspoons), in a tightly covered vessel, boiling water (1 pint), allowing to stand half an hour, straining with pressure, passing water through strainer to make 1 pint; if activity of infusion (herb) is affected by heat, only cold water should be used; the strength of infusions of energetic or powerful herbs should be specially directed by a physician or practitioner. A regular cup of tea is an infusion.

Inhalations, Vapors

Volatile liquid vapors breathed at ordinary inhalation, to act locally upon the respiratory mucous membrane.

Injections, Injectiones

Usually aqueous solutions of vegetable herbs to be injected by a syringe into the rectum (enemas), under the skin (hypodermic), or into the urethral, nasal, aural, or vaginal tract.

Insufflations

Fine powders of active medicine, and mostly bland bases, to be blown into nose, larynx, throat, and so on.

Inunctions

Medicated ointments containing hydrous wool fat, 85 to 95 percent.

Iodine

Iodine is a nonmetallic element with a metallic luster of a crimson-purplish color. It is found in cod-liver oil, shellfish, and most marine plants. Foods containing the most iodine are artichokes, asparagus, bananas, carrots, egg yolk, garlic, leeks, melons, mushrooms, onions, peas, spinach, and watercress. Herbs which contain high levels of iodine are kelp, dulse, and Irish moss.

The cells of the body which collect the by-products of cellular metabolism, called phagocytes, require iodine to function properly. The brain cells and nervous system also require sufficient iodine to perform at optimum efficiency. Iodine enables the tissues of muscles to store oxygen, and burns up food and prevents formation of fats. Chlorine speeds up the loss of iodine from the body. This should be noted by anyone engaged in water sports and those whose drinking water has been treated with chlorine (many city supplies are thus treated).

Iodine is extremely toxic in its pure form. Tincture of iodine (a 2 or 3 percent solution in alcohol) is used externally as an antiseptic for cuts, scratches, and bruises. It is taken internally in the form of Lugol's solution (a strong solution of iodine, potassium, iodide, and water) under medical supervision to treat several conditions, including poliomyelitis, tuberculosis, certain nutritional disorders, some forms of ovarian cysts, syphilis, and in disorders of the thyroid gland, which is where the body produces iodine for its own utilization.

Ions (Ionization)

Intense electrical activity occurring at the edge of the earth's atmosphere causes a breakdown of oxygen in a process caused by the ultraviolet rays of the sun. This is called ionization, which produces a layer of positively and negatively charged particles which make up the "ionosphere." Throughout millennia, this protective layer has built up, and its presence protects humans from receiving excessive, harmful amounts of ultraviolet rays from the sun. Some of these negative-charged ions filter down through the layers of the atmosphere and accumulate in various places such as the seashore and where there are waterfalls. The concentrations of the positive ions are felt to be detrimental to human health, and negative ions are felt to have a beneficial effect.

Medical researchers have discovered that exposing a person to quantities of negative ionic particles speeds up the healing process. Thus this method is employed in cases of severe burns, insomnia, and certain mental illnesses. Equipment to produce concentrations of negative ionization is usually quite expensive and is sometimes used by charlatans to offer speedy cures in dubious circumstances for absurdly high fees.

Iridology: Iris Diagnosis

The science of iridology had its beginnings in the middle of the nineteenth century in Budapest, Hungary. In the 1820s, Ignatz von Peckzely of Budapest was a small boy fascinated with birds. By chance, one day he caught an owl, and, in the struggle to subdue it, the owl's right leg was broken. As Peckzely later recalled, he noticed on looking into the owl's wide eyes after the injury to the limb that a small black spot had formed in the otherwise clear eye.

He prepared a splint, repaired the leg, and kept the bird for a pet. During the healing of the leg, Peckzely noticed that the black spot in the eye became coated with a white film and surrounded by a white border. He later realized that this denoted formation of scar tissue.

Peckzely was imprisoned in 1848 for revolutionary activities; this gave him ample time to pursue his hobby of examining eyes and to develop his theory that injuries leave visible signs in the eyes. He became more and more certain about the discovery with the owl in his childhood. When he was released from prison, he took a post as an intern (he was a lay practitioner) in the surgical wards of a college hospital, where he had an opportunity to observe many thousands of patients before and after accidents and operations. It was from viewing these changes that he was able to prepare a chart of the eyes. In 1866, he began practicing medicine in Budapest and published his first book on the iris, *Discovery in the Realm of Nature and Art of Healing.* At about the same time, the Swedish homeopath Nils Liljequist made practically identical discoveries about the iris and brought the work to America.

In the United States and Great Britain, others have further developed and expanded Peckzely's pioneering work. Among the physicians who have contributed to the science of iridology are Lindlahr, Dritzer, Boyd, Brown-Neil, Lahn, Francis, and Jensen.

Theory of Iridology

Every organ and part of the body is represented in a well-defined area in the iris. The nerve filaments, muscle fibers, and minute blood vessels in these areas of the iris react to changing conditions in the corresponding organs with visible signs such as spots, lines, lesions, and changes in pigment density. By means of these various marks, signs, and discolorations in the iris, nature reveals inherited weaknesses and tendencies to ailments such as diabetes, tuberculosis, and so forth. Nature also reveals by such means acute or chronic catarrhal conditions, destruction of tissue, drug poisonings, broken bones, and surgical operations. From the eye, according to the science of iridology, one can read the general body condition and the state of every organ in the body. Signs of prolonged emotion and stress are also recorded. Furthermore, one skilled in iris diagnosis can predict the healing crises through which the body must pass on its way to health.

Diagnosis from the eye confirms Samuel Hahnemann's teaching that all acute diseases have a constitutional background of hereditary deficiencies. Finally, it reveals the gradual purification of the system of morbid matter and readjustment to normal conditions.

The diagram shows where all the vital organs and parts of the body are represented in various areas of the iris.

Body Conditions Shown in the Iris

An irritation in the body is transmitted through nerves, which stimulate a rush of blood, causing swelling and congestion. This is transmitted through reflex nerve stimulation to the corresponding area in the iris.

For diagnostic purposes, the umbilicus is the center of the body. This corresponds to the black pupil in the center of the iris. The chart shows the stomach as corresponding to the first circle surrounding the pupil. If dark lines or spots appear in this ring, it denotes gastric trouble. All medicines that show themselves in the iris are poisonous to the body.

The different colors representing certain drugs (such as red for iodine or greenish-yellow for quinine) found in the iris are created by pigments deposited in the surface layers of the iris.

In a similar manner, areas are marked on the chart to show the intestinal tract, pancreas, sympathetic nervous system, reproductive and urinary organs, and so forth.

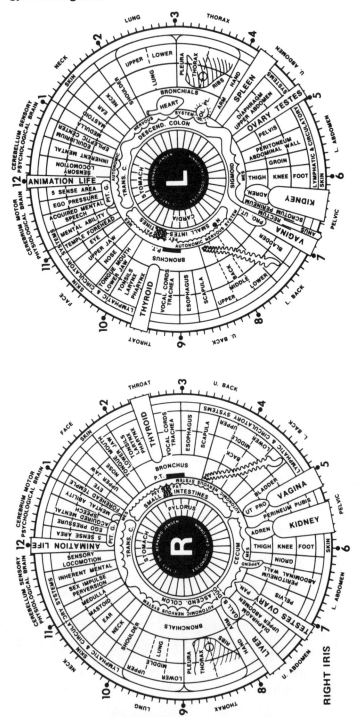

This iridology chart, developed by Dr. Bernard Jensen, shows the organ correspondence for all parts of the body.

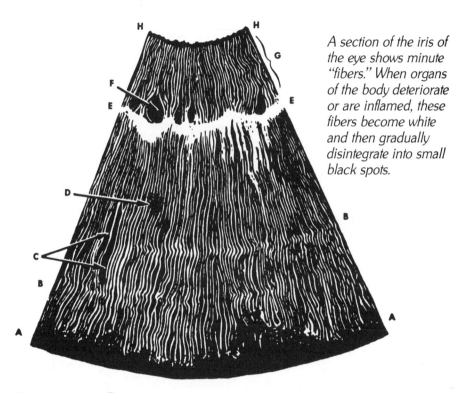

A section of the iris of the eye shows minute "fibers." When organs of the body deteriorate or are inflamed, these fibers become white and then gradually disintegrate into small black spots.

Development of Disease

The eye records three stages in the development of disease: acute, chronic, and destructive. The acute stage is the inflammatory condition, characterized by swelling, redness, heat, and pain. The chronic stage is also called the stage of failure. The acute stage occurs gradually and is shown in the iris by grayish-white lines. If drugs are used to check the acute stage, dark lines appear.

In the first, or acute, stage, tendencies to disease or weakness are shown by color, density, and hereditary lesion. The *color* indicates whether the tissues are normal or affected by disease. The *density* is the grain or structure composing the iris and gives information about the tone and vitality of the body. *Hereditary lesions* show as dull gray and indicate corresponding weaknesses in the same organs in the parent's body, unless they are due to recessive genes.

The chronic stage, marked by lowered vitality and pathogenic organisms in the system, gradually causes destruction of tissue. Similar changes take place in the areas of the iris; in these areas, the tissues dry, shrivel, and turn black. When this happens, the white signs of the acute states are intermingled with black streaks. In the advanced stage of destruction, the corresponding layers of the iris will be destroyed and leave a black spot.

Colors of the Iris

In a newborn Caucasian child, the iris is nearly always blue. This is because pigmentation develops after birth, and so the color of the eyes may alter. Colors vary in many types of people, but in Caucasians there are only two true iris pigments: light azure blue and light hazel brown. Non-Caucasians' eyes are dark brown or black. Other colors are really shades of these pigments. Color changes often occur in the iris, and these reflect the changing conditions of the person's health. Color spots indicate accumulations of drugs, taken either internally or externally. This shows that drugs are not always eliminated from the body, and because of their constant irritation, they can be factors in disease. Homeopathic remedies will not show in the iris, which demonstrates that they are nonpoisonous.

The Practice of Iridology

The practitioner of the science of iridology will use several terms to indicate symptoms: the *sympathetic wreath* shows the condition of the gastrointestinal tract; *nerve* or *cramp rings* indicate an overstimulation of the nervous system; white flakes in the outer rim of the iris are called *lymphatic rosary* and show inflammation of the lymph vessels; a scurf rim on the outermost rim of the iris shows poor condition of the skin; the *antonymis nerve wreath* shows the state of the nervous system; and the *psora* indicate internal lesions and possible tumor sites.

Generally speaking, the examiner will seat the patient in a comfortable chair and use an eye light with a small magnifying glass. He or she surveys the iris for color, overacidity, scurf rim, nerve rings, drug signs, acute signs, chronic signs, destructive signs, sympathetic wreath, and other factors. In some clinics, 35-millimeter slides are taken of the iris and then projected onto a large screen, and the signs are explained to the patient. Iridology practitioners do not prescribe treatment for specific diseases unless they are licensed in one of the healing arts.

It takes considerable instruction and practice to become proficient at reading the iris. The only tools needed are a small penlight and a 10X magnifying lens. In time, the layperson can develop the needed skill in reading her or his own and others' irises. More and more drugless physicians are relying on iris diagnosis, and while the science is still in its infancy, the results so far are remarkable.

Recently an Iridologist International Association has been formed to coordinate research and practice in the field of professional iridology. They have made their own iridology chart and can supply names of iridologists in the United States. The address is: Iridologists International, Route 1, Box 52, Escondido, Calif. 92025.

Iron *(Ferrum)*

A metal possessing a color from silver-white to gray, iron is taken internally as a component of various foods and is responsible for the red color of hemoglobin, a combination of iron and protein in the blood. The total amount of iron in the body at any time is usually not more than three to five grams. While most vitamins and nutrients are expended by the body, iron is stored and reused.

Low levels of iron are indicative of anemia, commonly caused by loss of blood from traumatic injury or excessive bleeding. Other causes of anemia are often due to the fact that the iron consumed is not being absorbed into the body. Iron occurs in two forms—ferrous and ferric. It is only the ferrous form that the body utilizes. Iron must also be combined with another substance, often copper, which renders it as a salt form—the only form in which the body can absorb it. In addition, there must be adequate hydrochloric acid present in the stomach and vitamin C in the bloodstream.

The best way to obtain adequate intake of iron is through foods. Foods that are rich sources of iron include asparagus, barley, blackstrap molasses, bran, dates, dried fruits, eggs, figs, lentils, lettuce, oats, olives, prunes, radishes, rye, walnuts, watercress, and wheat germ. The daily requirement of iron in the diet is usually given as 15 to 30 milligrams.

Iscador

An injectable made from mistletoe, developed by the Society for Cancer Research, Kirschweg 9, Arlesheim, Switzerland. The cost varies according to the type of iscador used, the frequency of injections, and the supplemental medication (to help the liver, bowels, and kidneys excrete the waste products) which may or may not be used.

Lucas Klinik, a medical clinic at Arlesheim, Switzerland, uses iscador, herbs with organic food, and so on, for treating cancer and other degenerative diseases, apparently with considerable success.

Isometrics

Developed as a military set of exercises to be done in confined quarters, isometric principles of exercise are now used by many people living a sedentary life, as they can be done while sitting and without any special equipment. The principle is to apply constant pressure, equal and opposite, on a muscle by such means as clenching and unclenching the fist or making circular arcs with the neck to develop muscle tone without working up a sweat. It is a worthwhile technique for those who are unable to engage in any other form of exercise.

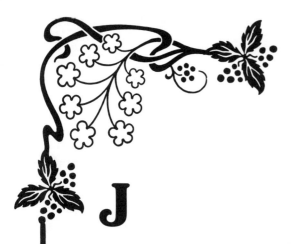

J

Jalap *(Exogonium purga)*

Its medicinal properties come from two resins, jalapin and convolvulin. Jalap is primarily a cathartic and chologogue, and also used to eliminate large amounts of water from the body. To reduce fever and inflammations, a combination of 1 teaspoon each of jalap and calomel is often used. For children, ⅛ teaspoon of jalap tea is mixed with syrup of rhubarb to accomplish the same purpose. Jalap also acts to expel worms. Use of jalap is not recommended when there is inflammation of the intestinal mucous membrane. If the resin is used, the dose is a few grains (less than ⅛ of a teaspoon).

Jethro Kloss Therapy (See *Kloss, Jethro*)

Jujube

A preparation obtainable from Eastern pharmacies, made from a species of dates. An acceptable substitute is made by mixing equal parts of gum arabic and turbinado sugar, or honey.

Juniper *(Juniperus communis)*

The fruit of *Juniperus communis* contains a volatile oil which is a stomachic, a tonic, a diuretic, and an aphrodisiac. The kidneys act to eliminate the oil, and thus juniper is often employed in cystitis and similar afflictions. A tar from the tree is also used in many skin conditions. In cases of feverous diseases or inflammation, a decoction of the berries is made by softening the skins in 1 pint of water for one-half hour, draining, and then pouring 1 pint of boiling water over the berries for one-half hour or more. A ½-teacup portion is consumed after meals and at bedtime.

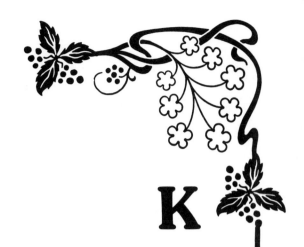

K

K Vitamin

Vitamin K, known as the clotting factor, was discovered in 1934 by the Danish researcher Henrik Dam during his studies on artificial hemorrhaging diseases of birds. Vitamin K is necessary for production in the liver of prothrombin and other blood-clotting factors, which can be reduced to pathologically low levels if enough Vitamin K is not consumed for several months.

Humans and most other animals can survive without foods containing this vitamin, because the bacteria in the liver will synthesize prothrombin in adequate amounts. However, as vitamin K is fat-soluble, if the bile, liver, or lymph is malfunctioning, manufacture of vitamin K is suspended. Vitamin K is often given to counteract possible slow blood clotting before surgery for obstruction of the ducts of the gall bladder or liver.

Vitamin K is found in large amounts in alfalfa and is also synthesized and sold commercially. Foods rich in vitamin K are all salad greens, spinach, and green cabbage.

Vitamin K is very unstable and sensitive to light, and thus should be stored in amber containers, away from direct light.

Kapferer System

Dr. Richard Kapferer, although greatly influenced by his contemporary, Father Sebastian Kneipp (1821–1897), was responsible for bringing considerable scientific evaluation to the medical application of fasting. His method involved continuing a fast for as long as necessary to effect complete internal cleansing; many nature-cure doctors prescribed only short fasts.

Kefir

A fermented drink made from cow's milk, to which is added a ferment taken from a mushroom found growing in the Caucasus Mountains. Asiatic natives use it as a remedy for anemia, lung disorders, and stomach diseases. The following chart shows the composition of kefir and cow's milk.

	Cow's Milk	Kefir
albuminoids (casein, etc.)	4%	4%
butter	4	2
sugar of milk	5	2
lactic acid		1
alcohol		1
water and salt	87	90

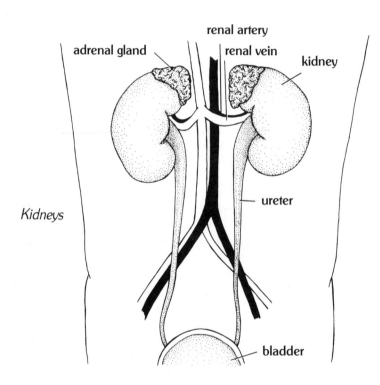

Kidneys

Kidneys

The kidneys are two paired organs situated in the back part of the abdominal cavity, one on each side of the spinal column. The right kidney is usually somewhat lower than the left. In the adult, each kidney is approximately 4 inches high and 2 inches long, and weighs from 4½ to 6 ounces. They extend from the twelfth dorsal to the third lumbar vertebra.

The kidneys are covered by a sheath of connective tissue called the capsule of the kidney. The functional units of the kidneys are nephrons; there are about one million of these small tubes in each kidney. They collect the waste products of the kidneys—water, carbon dioxide, salts, and urea—which are eliminated in the urine. Another small tube, called a ureter, is connected to each side of the kidney, and through these ducts urine is conveyed to the bladder for elimination.

Kinesiology (Applied Kinesiology)

Kinesiology is the science of the mechanics and anatomy of muscles and muscle movement. Applied kinesiology relates various muscle weaknesses to symptoms of diseases.

The development of applied kinesiology as a science is credited to Dr. George Goodheart, presently director of research at the International College of Applied Kinesiology in Detroit, Michigan. In 1965, quite by accident, he discovered a correlation between a patient's disease symptoms and corresponding weakness of a muscle. By trial and error, he worked out the first charting of the reflexes of muscles and the corresponding organs of the entire body. He developed a systematic method of considering a patient as being influenced by the "Triad of Health," with the mind, body, and spirit forming the pyramid.

If a patient comes to a practitioner of applied kinesiology, and a series of "muscle tests" finds muscles or sets of muscles weak, then the corresponding organ is thought to be malfunctioning. Nutrition, manipulation, and acupressure meridians are all employed, singly or in combination, in the pathway to health.

Applied kinesiology is learned in a hundred-hour course at any facility approved by the International College of Applied Kinesiology (ICAK.) An additional three hundred hours of instruction qualifies a practitioner to become a diplomate of the ICAK, after a rigorous examination. In 1978, there were less than a hundred diplomates in the United States, due to the strict requirements for education and practice.

Lay practitioners of applied kinesiology abound in most cities. Many of these people learned the rudiments of the science from seminars or as part of a curriculum in a natural-healing college. *Touch for Health,* by Dr. John Thie and Mary Marks (Marina del Rey, Calif.: DeVorss, 1979), is widely used by lay practitioners, as it provides understandable information and instruction on basic anatomy, muscle functions, nutrition, diagrams of the meridian system of acupressure, and maps of the various "reflex points" in the body.

Professional athletes and their trainers also utilize the principles of applied kinesiology, with some adherents claiming to have set new records in various sports after employing this program of muscle testing and building.

Kino

The inspissated juice of *Pterocarpus marsupium,* a plant native to India, kino is used in tincture form as an ingredient in gargles and medicines for diarrhea. The dose of the tincture is ½ teaspoon.

Kloss, Jethro

Author of the now-famous book on nature cure *Back to Eden* (Woodbridge Press Publishing Co., Santa Barbara, Cal., 1975). Jethro Kloss (1863–1946) was one of the early pioneers of herbal medicine in the United States. Relying on his own use of diet and herbs to recover from various diseases as a young man, he practiced successfully as a lay doctor for most of his adult life. The cornerstone of his philosophy was, "Revolutionize the common manner of living, eating and drinking, and you will have a happier and healthier people."

Back to Eden is a compendium of Kloss's experience with diets, water cure, fasting, massage, enemas, and the application of herbs to a wide variety of illnesses. A cancer-cure regimen known as the Jethro Kloss Therapy is summed up as follows: "Correct food, herbs, water, fresh air, massage, sunshine, exercise and rest."

Among the herbs he recommended for cancer were violet leaves, red clover blossoms, burdock root, yellow dock root, golden seal root, gum myrrh, echinecea, aloes, cayenne, rock rose, and Oregon grape.

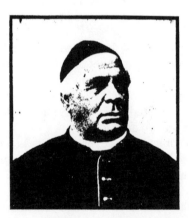

Father Sebastian Kneipp (1821-1897) cured himself of a lung condition by swimming in ice-cold water. His rapid recovery led him to develop a system of cold-water therapeutics, which is still used in many parts of Europe and the United States.

Kneipp Water Therapy

Use of water as a therapeutic agent was advanced into a scientific modality in modern times by Sebastian Kneipp (1821–1897). Afflicted with a presumably fatal lung condition, Father Kneipp studied the medical writings of Vincenz

Priessnitz and healed himself by plunging into ice-cold water every day for many months. He fully recovered his health, and as a result, developed a water-cure system which utilized not only ice-cold baths, but also walking barefoot in grass and cold streams. His curative system further developed and included the use of herbs, light, and fresh air.

The Kneipp water cure became so famous that twenty thousand patients came to his clinic annually, but since he was a priest and not a physician, medical doctors never came to rely upon his system. The Kneipp water cure is still widely practiced in Germany, Austria, and Switzerland.

Kombé (See *Strophanthus, Kombé*)

Krebiozen and Carcalon

Krebiozen is a nontoxic local tissue hormone, or "tissue autacoid," used for cancer treatment and administered by injection, which was discovered by Dr. Stevan Durovic, a Yugoslavian who came to the United States in 1949. Andrew C. Ivy, M.D., a distinguished Professor Emeritus of physiology and retired vice-president and head of the medical school at the University of Illinois, was a leading sponsor of Krebiozen, which is now apparently unavailable. Dr. Ivy authored or coauthored more than fifteen hundred scientific articles and was regarded by many as the world's greatest living physiologist.

Dr. Ivy's own discovery, Carcalon, is an injectable which is somewhat more effective than Krebiozen for cancer.

Before the use of Krebiozen was discontinued, tumors were arrested or reduced in 86 percent of patients treated with it. Pain was improved in 62.6 percent and use of narcotics decreased or stopped in 48 percent of the patients. About five hundred of the first four thousand patients classed as 98 percent "hopeless" who received Krebiozen recovered according to reports gathered from three thousand doctors.

The Food and Drug Administration (FDA) banned the drug from interstate commerce in July 1963. As a result of the FDA's decision to prevent willing doctors from giving willing patients a safe substance, a joint resolution (cosponsored by seventeen senators and thirty-nine representatives) was introduced in Congress which would have directed the FDA to lift the ban until the completion of a fair test by the National Cancer Institute. The sponsors, however, could not muster sufficient support and the bill died.

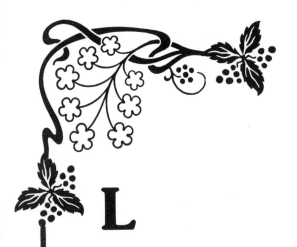

L

Lactation (See *Infant Feeding*)

Lactic Acid Fermentation Diet

An adjunctive method of treating and preventing cancer and other chronic diseases with diet and medicines, developed by Johannes Kuhl of West Germany, a professor at the Nuclear Research Institute at Rome, Italy. His lactic acid bread, lactic acid butter, lactic acid soured vegetables, and so on may not yet be available in English-speaking countries. (Check your health food store for other lactic acid fermented products.) According to Professor Kuhl, "the lactic acid milk products (sour cream milk, buttermilk, butter-milk curds) are a valuable diet food only in connection with an unleavened vegetable food." Using lactic acid milk products only is not felt to be a valuable diet nourishment.

Dr. Kuhl's lactic acid fermented plant concentrate (from egg white and Indian corn), called Viscolaticum, is very helpful, as are lactic acid fermented wheat and lactic acid fermented muesli (a cereal). These can be prepared at home (except for the Viscolaticum), and the muesli can become a permanent addition to one's diet.

The Viscolaticum is used to prevent and treat increased pathological fermentation in tissues that results from dysoxidation in cells caused by chronically increased glycolytic splitting. It acts to normalize cell respiration, which is subnormal in all acute and chronic conditions.

The fermenting wheat and muesli grow valuable molds (such as rhizopus, mucorales, penicillin, and different types of aspergillales) that make their own natural vitamins (including the whole B complex), hormones, enzymes, cell activators and regulators, as well as powerful, natural antibiotics, all free of harmful side effects. This is preventative and curative dietary therapy against serious acute, chronic, and infectious diseases, including malignancies, Hodgkin's disease, multiple sclerosis, stomach and intestinal disorders, and climacterial and prostate conditions.

The diet also balances defective nutrition, corrects calcium deficiency (rick-

ets) in children, and protects against the deposition of strontium 90 (a dangerous radioactive fallout) in the bones and bone marrow.

For details about Dr. Kuhl's therapy, read *Checkmate for Cancer* by Viad-
rina Vertag and A. Trowitzch (Broulage, Harzburger Str. G, West Germany).

Laetrile (Nitriloside)

A nontoxic compound (occurring in 1200 natural foods), generally administered by injection, which breaks down into benzaldehyde, glucuronic acid
and hydrocyanic acid in the body. The chemical name is laevo-mandelonitri-
lebeta glucuronoside. The generic term is *amygdalin,* which *Webster's New
Collegiate Dictionary* describes as: "a white crystalline cyanogenetic glucoside . . . found . . . in the bitter almond." Its use as a cancer treatment was
developed by Ernst T. Krebs, Sr., M.D., and his son, Dr. Ernst T. Krebs, Jr.,
who heads the John Beard Memorial Foundation (P.O. Box 685, San Francisco, Calif. 94101). Ernesto Contreras, M.D., in Tijuana, Mexico, gives the
treatment (P.O. Box 3793, San Ysidro, Calif. 92073).

The prognosis for cancer therapy with Laetrile after prior treatment with
radiation is often poor, since radiation burns up the capillaries needed to carry
the Laetrile to the cancer cells. Laetrile liberates hydrocyanic acid in the tumor
(not in the healthy cells, where the enzyme rhodanase neutralizes the Laetrile)
and kills tumor respiration. Most tumors contain sufficient amounts of the enzyme beta-glucoronidase to "trigger off" the cyanide in the tumor from the
Laetrile. If Laetrile alone has no effect, then the clinician also injects the beta-
glucoronidase—but not with, immediately before, or immediately after using
Laetrile.

In those cases where drainage is inadequate or detoxification and excretion
are impaired, products of tumor breakdown will not be eliminated readily. In
such situations, high dosage may be followed by toxemia.

On the basis of present knowledge, it is felt that the average cancer case
requires a total of three hundred grams of Laetrile to reach the point where oral
maintenance dosages are sufficient.

Although Laetrile has been used with good results since the 1920s and is
now used in fourteen countries, it has been banned from interstate commerce
in the United States by the Food and Drug Administration. As this is written,
Laetrile can be used legally by doctors in California, Arizona, and Indiana.

Lakhovsky Multiwave Oscillator

The principle behind this therapeutic device was developed by Georges Lakhovsky, a Russian engineer who emigrated to France in the 1930s. His idea
was that all matter, organic and inorganic, vibrates and sends off a specific
frequency. All animals, vegetables, and minerals have their specific frequencies
and, furthermore, each organ within the body has a specific vibratory rate.

Lakhovsky invented a machine, quite large and expensive due to its complexity, which was able to create these oscillatory fields. By turning the device to the specific frequency of a particular organ, for example, the person undergoing exposure experienced therapeutic effects.

Generally speaking, a patient is seated between two electrodes and the current is passed through the body. The multiwave oscillator thus provides the two poles of vibration—one generative and the other resonant—and as the current passes through living tissue, the affected organ is restored to its most balanced, or properly healthy rhythm.

For a time, Lakhovsky's Multiwave Oscillator was considered a fraudulent device used only by quacks. Additional research by many scientists, including Andrevont and Shereshevsky of Harvard University, later conclusively proved the value of Lakhovsky's theory. Nevertheless, although transistors have made production of the device economically feasible today and the theory is sound, few practitioners use it. The idea behind oscillatory therapy—that each cell is capable of transmitting and receiving radiation—is also the basis of radionic diagnosis. (See also *Radiesthesia*.)

It may eventually be proved that the ability of mystics and psychics to heal over great distances, without being physically present with a patient, is due to the ability of these oscillatory waves to travel over great distances, as do radio and other waves.

Large Intestine

The large intestine, also called the colon, extends from the small intestine to the anus and is ordinarily about 5 feet in length. The topmost part of the colon is called the *cecum*. On its lower end, there is protrusion about 4 inches long called the *veriform appendix,* which is thought to be a vestigial organ.

The large intestine is divided into three parts: ascending, transverse, and descending. At the top of the pelvis, the colon makes a curve downward at the juncture known as the *sigmoid flexure.* From this point on, the colon is known as the *rectum,* a section about 6 inches in length terminating at the anus, which is the opening for emitting waste matters. The anus is controlled by reflexive muscles called the *sphincters.*

The main functions of the large intestine are absorption of water and elimination of waste products. The fluid secreted by the large intestine is thick and full of mucus. Foreign substances, including drugs, are eliminated by the large intestine. Large numbers of bacteria are usually consumed with food. Most of these are destroyed by the sterilizing and digestive action of the acids of the stomach, but some pass through unaffected and appear in the large intestine.

The principal changes brought about by bacteria in the intestines are fermentations. Proteins are also acted upon, giving rise to a number of putrefactive gases (H_2S, H_2, CO_2 and CH_4), volatile acids, and amines. These gases are primarily responsible for the characteristic odor of feces.

Some of the amines are toxic but usually have no effect upon the body, for even if they are reabsorbed, they are rendered harmless by the detoxifying action of the liver.

If the intestinal putrefaction is excessive, if the mucus is hard and thick, or if the liver is weak and degenerated, toxic products of digestion may enter the general bloodstream and produce toxic effects.

Larynx

The larynx is made up of muscular, membranous, and cartilage tissue and is the primary organ which produces the voice. It is located in the upper part of the throat between the trachea and the base of the tongue. In the upper, forward part of the neck, this cartilage forms the protrusion known as the Adam's Apple.

Lavage

Washing out the stomach is sometimes required for diagnostic or therapeutic purposes, including the removal of mucus, acids, poisons, and so forth. The method usually employed is to insert a soft rubber tube into the stomach through the mouth and down the throat. The tube is about 3 feet long, with a bulb on one end and a funnel attached for pouring in pure water.

Lavage is most frequently performed before breakfast or long after eating a meal. The patient is seated in a low chair and the tube is passed down the esophagus while the patient is encouraged to say ahhh, to aid in opening the throat. Enough warm water—about a pint—is then introduced into the tube until it backs up in the funnel, at which time the water collected in the stomach will run out the funnel into a basin held by or for the patient.

Lavage should always be performed under a doctor's supervision.

Lavatio

Mouthwashes of soap dissolved in 75 percent colored water and flavored with essential oils to please; antiseptic, purifier.

Lavender *(Lavandula vera)*

The flowers of *Lavandula vera* derive their medicinal value from the presence of a volatile oil. It is aromatic, stimulant, carminative, and used also in flavorings and as a medium or agent for giving other medicines. One to 5 drops of the oil are used, or 10 drops of the tincture.

Laxatives

Constipation is often found in conjunction with chronic and degenerative diseases. While there is no hard-and-fast rule for the proper number of bowel movements each day, most physicians would agree that two movements per day are ordinary for healthy people.

While there are many herbs, spices, and teas which produce laxative effects, the use of foods high in cellulose, or "bulk," are thought to aid regular bowel movements. Among those foods which help accomplish this purpose are the following:

apples	grapes	prunes
beet-top greens	green peas	raisins
bran	lettuce	spinach
buttermilk	mustard greens	string beans
cabbage, raw	oatmeal	tomatoes
carrots	oranges	turnips
cauliflower	parsnips	whole wheat
celery	peaches	
dandelion greens	pears	
grapefruit	plums	

Lecithin

A phosphorized fat found in nerve tissue, egg yolk, and in some quantity in almost all animal and vegetable cells. Nutritionists think it assists the metabolizing of food substances and is utilized to prevent malnutrition in bottle-fed infants. Many as-yet unverified nutritional claims have been made for the substance.

Leeching

The withdrawing of blood by means of blood sucking worms has been practiced in healing for thousands of years. In the United States, leeching has dwindled to a rarely used folk remedy for black eyes, and leeches are available from only one commercial source at the present.

In the humoral medicine of the East, application of leeches is recommended in many conditions of inflammation and to withdraw "infected" blood from various sites.

The method used is to first clean the area thoroughly with soap and water. If the area is contaminated, especially with liniments or salves, the leeches will refuse to take hold and bite. Sometimes a drop of blood or milk is put in the skin where the leech is to be applied.

The incision of the leech is made by razor-sharp teeth, which puncture the skin without pain. Medicinal leeches available in the United States are imported from Poland and are of the species *Huris medicinalis.*

A leech will extract approximately ½ to 1 ounce of blood per treatment, and since each leech can live up to twelve months on one feeding, additional leeches must be procured if the treatment is to be repeated.

The wound is likely to continue bleeding after the leech is removed. The application of a little table salt to the leech will ordinarily cause it to drop off. Stopping of blood flow can be effected by applying a sterile pad with pressure for a few minutes. Leeches should not be applied to delicate or "loose" skin, on the eyes, or to genital parts without medical supervision.

Licorice Root (*Glycyrrhiza glabra*)

The root of *G. glabra* is a demulcent and mild laxative with a sweetish taste. It is often employed as an excipient in pills and lozenges. Other principal preparations are as a tea, an extract, a fluidextract, and compounded with other herbs.

Licorice has been prescribed since the time of Hippocrates for a variety of ailments, including dropsy, coughs, sore throats, and catarrhal conditions of the urinary tract.

The dosage of the powdered root is ½ to 1 teaspoon, as a tea.

Licorice is also used by brewers to impart the deep, dark color and flavor to stout beers, and in the manufacture of tobacco for smoking and chewing.

Life Expectancy

The following table provides statistical data on the average number of years Americans can expect to live.

Commissioners 1958 Standard Ordinary Mortality Table

Age	Number Living	Deaths Each Year	Deaths per 1,000	Average Future Lifetime
0	10,000,000	70,800	7.08	68.30
1	9,929,200	17,475	1.76	67.78
2	9,911,725	15,066	1.52	66.90
3	9,896,659	14,449	1.46	66.00

Age	Number Living	Deaths Each Year	Deaths per 1,000	Average Future Lifetime
4	9,882,210	13,835	1.40	65.10
5	9,868,375	13,322	1.35	64.19
6	9,855,053	12,812	1.30	63.27
7	9,842,241	12,401	1.26	62.35
8	9,829,840	12,091	1.23	61.43
9	9,817,749	11,879	1.21	60.51
10	9,805,870	11,865	1.21	59.58
11	9,794,005	12,047	1.23	58.65
12	9,781,958	12,325	1.26	57.72
13	9,769,633	12,896	1.32	56.80
14	9,756,737	13,562	1.39	55.87
15	9,743,175	14,225	1.46	54.95
16	9,728,950	14,983	1.54	54.03
17	9,713,967	15,737	1.62	53.11
18	9,698,230	16,390	1.69	52.19
19	9,681,840	16,846	1.74	51.28
20	9,664,994	17,300	1.79	50.37
21	9,647,694	17,655	1.83	49.46
22	9,630,039	17,912	1.86	48.55
23	9,612,127	18,167	1.89	47.64
24	9,593,960	18,324	1.91	46.73
25	9,575,636	18,481	1.93	45.82
26	9,557,155	18,732	1.96	44.90
27	9,538,423	18,981	1.99	43.99
28	9,519,442	19,324	2.03	43.08
29	9,500,118	19,760	2.08	42.16
30	9,480,358	20,193	2.13	41.25
31	9,460,165	20,718	2.19	40.34
32	9,439,447	21,239	2.25	39.43
33	9,418,208	21,850	2.32	38.51
34	9,396,358	22,551	2.40	37.60
35	9,373,807	23,528	2.51	36.69
36	9,350,279	24,685	2.64	35.78
37	9,325,594	26,112	2.80	34.88
38	9,299,482	27,991	3.01	33.97
39	9,271,491	30,132	3.25	33.07
40	9,241,359	32,622	3.53	32.18
41	9,208,737	35,362	3.84	31.29
42	9,173,375	38,253	4.17	30.41

Age	Number Living	Deaths Each Year	Deaths per 1,000	Average Future Lifetime
43	9,135,122	41,382	4.53	29.54
44	9,093,740	44,741	4.92	28.67
45	9,048,999	48,412	5.35	27.81
46	9,000,587	52,473	5.83	26.95
47	8,948,114	56,910	6.36	26.11
48	8,891,204	61,794	6.95	25.27
49	8,829,410	67,104	7.60	24.45
50	8,762,306	72,902	8.32	23.63
51	8,689,404	79,160	9.11	22.82
52	8,610,244	85,758	9.96	22.03
53	8,524,486	92,832	10.89	21.25
54	8,431,654	100,337	11.90	20.47
55	8,331,317	108,307	13.00	19.71
56	8,223,010	116,849	14.21	18.97
57	8,106,161	125,970	15.54	18.23
58	7,980,191	135,663	17.00	17.51
59	7,844,528	145,830	18.59	16.81
60	7,698,698	156,592	20.34	16.12
61	7,542,106	167,736	22.24	15.44
62	7,374,370	179,271	24.31	14.78
63	7,195,099	191,174	26.57	14.14
64	7,003,925	203,394	29.04	13.51
65	6,800,531	215,917	31.75	12.90
66	6,584,614	228,749	34.74	12.31
67	6,355,865	241,777	38.04	11.73
68	6,114,088	254,835	41.68	11.17
69	5,859,253	267,241	45.61	10.64
70	5,592,012	278,426	49.79	10.12
71	5,313,586	287,731	54.15	9.63
72	5,025,855	294,766	58.65	9.15
73	4,731,089	299,289	63.26	8.69
74	4,431,800	301,894	68.12	8.24
75	4,129,906	303,011	73.37	7.81
76	3,826,895	303,014	79.18	7.39
77	3,523,881	301,997	85.70	6.98
78	3,221,884	299,829	93.06	6.59
79	2,922,055	295,683	101.19	6.21
80	2,626,372	288,848	109.98	5.85

81	2,337,524	278,983	119.35	5.51
82	2,058,541	265,902	129.17	5.19
83	1,792,639	249,858	139.38	4.89
84	1,542,781	231,433	150.01	4.60
85	1,311,348	211,311	161.14	4.32
86	1,100,037	190,108	172.82	4.06
87	909,929	168,455	185.13	3.80
88	741,474	146,997	198.25	3.55
89	594,477	126,303	212.46	3.31
90	468,174	106,809	228.14	3.06
91	361,365	88,813	245.77	2.82
92	272,552	72,480	265.93	2.58
93	200,072	57,881	289.30	2.33
94	142,191	45,026	316.66	2.07
95	97,165	34,128	351.24	1.80
96	63,037	25,250	400.56	1.51
97	37,787	18,456	488.42	1.18
98	19,331	12,916	668.15	.83
99	6,415	6,415	1,000.00	.50

Liniment

Also called a salve, a liniment is a thin, liquid ointment for external application, usually containing a quantity of medicinal oil. Typical liniments are those of belladonna, camphor, soap, turpentine, calcium, and so forth.

Linseed (Flaxseed) *Linum usitatissimum*

The seeds of *Linum usitatissimum* are cultivated annually for their demulcent, emollient, and expectorant properties. Perhaps its widest use is as a stomachic cleanser and to soothe inflammations of the intestinal tract and throat and urinary passages. A drop of the oil of flaxseed is used internally in cases of hemorrhoids. Poultices of linseed are applied to burns.

Liquors

Mostly aqueous solutions of nonvolatile chemical substances.

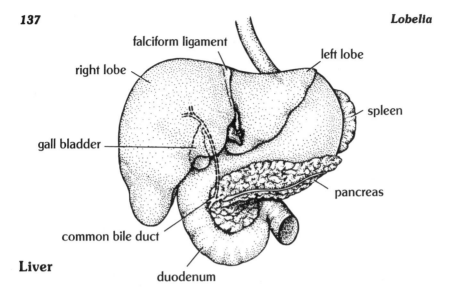

right lobe

falciform ligament

left lobe

spleen

gall bladder

pancreas

common bile duct

duodenum

Liver

The liver is a compound tubular gland located in the upper right part of the abdominal cavity, immediately below the diaphragm. It is the largest gland of the body, weighing about 1500 grams.

The main functions of the liver are secretion of bile, formation of blood, metabolism, detoxification, and a thermal function relating to temperature maintained. Some researchers believe that the liver can accomplish reoxidation and metabolic regeneration.

There are several thousand enzymes which have been identified as being manufactured in the liver and which often act as catalysts in remote parts of the body and other organs. While the full range of functions of the liver is just beginning to be understood, many researchers agree that the liver is the "wheel of life," whose functions can be compared with the function of chlorophyll in plants.

The humoral system of Eastern medicine and Hippocrates holds that the four humors (yellow and black bile, blood, and phlegm) arise in the liver. Thus most, if not all, treatments in Eastern medicine involve the liver directly.

Max Gerson, M.D., a pioneer in nontoxic cancer therapy, concluded that the recovery possibilities of cancer victims depend directly upon the degree of liver degeneration and damage (see *Gerson Therapy*). Since the liver has great functional reserves, and deterioration of liver function can be quite advanced before detection, it is difficult to determine when pathological destruction of the liver actually begins.

Lobelia

Of all the herbs in the United States used for healing purposes, perhaps *Lobelia inflata,* also known as Indian tobacco, has generated more controversy than any other. Its mention in herbal lore goes back centuries, but since it is native to the United States, it is not surprising that the main application of lobelia has occurred in the United States.

Samuel Thomson, a New Hampshire self-educated herbal doctor who lived in the late 1700s, discovered that lobelia was capable of generating a very intense internal heat and, if consumed in small, frequent doses, could raise a vigorous perspiration, after which a long sleep of ten to twelve hours followed. Upon waking, the patient was often either cured or greatly improved. During his lifetime, Thomson's system of herbal medicine was fairly reported to have been used effectively on more than two million persons.

Thomson was persecuted by orthodox medical practitioners, one of whom managed to have Thomson arrested for murder. The case was tried before the New York State Supreme Court, which acquitted Thomson even before he had to present a defense.

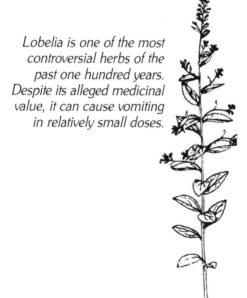

Lobelia is one of the most controversial herbs of the past one hundred years. Despite its alleged medicinal value, it can cause vomiting in relatively small doses.

Dr. Thomson wrote a fascinating autobiography of his medical discoveries, along with a complete description of his vegetable system of medicine. According to him, the entire supply of medicine for a family of eight would, even at today's prices, cost no more than a few dollars. Thomson's book, *Guide to Health,* published in 1825, has recently been reissued in an inexpensive reprint edition and is available from Health Research, Mokulemne Hills, Calif.

The leaves and tops of lobelia are used as an expectorant, a diaphoretic, a purgative, an antispasmodic and an emetic. In large doses, it is a motor depres-

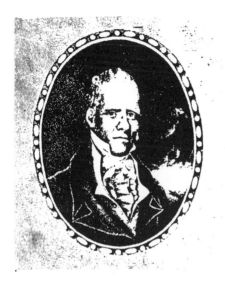

Samuel Thomson used lobelia as the basis of his system of natural healing. He is said to have cured more than 20 million persons in his lifetime with the "Thomsonian System." Lobelia is believed to stimulate the body's natural healing system by promoting a free and full perspiration, which carries toxins out of the system.

sant and somewhat narcotic. It is a specific for asthma and, in tincture form, a few drops in the mouth have been claimed to halt the spasms of seizures. The only identified active ingredient is an alkaloid, lobeline.

Today the Food and Drug Administration has labeled this herb unsafe, although it is still widely sold across the country. There has been some effort to grow it as a tenant farm crop in the southeastern United States.

Lotions

Mostly weak water medicinal solutions or mixtures to be applied locally with linen, lint, or muslin.

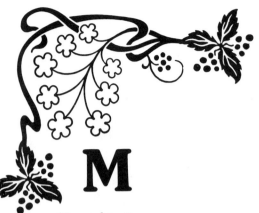

M

Macrobiotics

Coined by the Japanese author and teacher Georges Ohsawa, the term is derived from the Greek words *macro* ("large"), and *bio* ("life"). Ohsawa's *Zen Macrobiotics: The Art of Rejuvenation and Longevity,* first appeared in this country in 1962. Lectures and cooking classes given by Michio and Aveline Kushi, students of Ohsawa, served to disseminate information and practical application of the diet and its philosophical principles. At this time, there are centers of study all over the world and a main center for study in Boston, Massachusetts, where Mr. and Mrs. Kushi reside and teach.

The basis of the dietary regime is the principle of primary and secondary foods, the primary foods being whole grains and cereals and the secondary foods being vegetables from the land and sea. Also included are beans of various kinds, fermented products, seeds, and nuts and fruits in season.

How these foods are selected and prepared is the key to health, according to macrobiotic theory. An individual's "constitution," that is, the quality of his or her internal organs at birth, will determine to a large extent the kinds of food he or she will be attracted to. By understanding what our original constitution was, we can see why our present condition is what it is and take the proper dietary steps to correct the imbalances.

Ohsawa refers to the principles of "yin" and "yang" as a compass that points the direction in which an individual should go. With this yin and yang compass, a person should be able to judge his or her own actual needs and select the proper foods accordingly. Yin and yang are two poles or "arms" of infinity, according to Oriental cosmology, which interact with each other and create the universe and all phenomena. In order to make the diet more understandable, Ohsawa divided foods into yin and yang classification. For example:

Yin	Neutral	Yang	
chemicals	tomato	burdock	sea salt
refined sugar	spinach	onion	fish
honey	celery	carrot	poultry
fruit	cabbage	seaweed	dairy
potato	turnip	grains	meat

Yin and yang are also divided into opposites, such as night/day, expansion/ contraction, large/small, light/heavy, purple/red, cold/hot, and so on.

Macrobiotics teaches that since our blood has a ratio of 7 to 1 of potassium to sodium, we should eat as close to that ratio as possible. Tropical fruits, like banana which has a ratio of 800 to 1, are very difficult to assimilate, as is the high sodium content in animal products plus the quality of animal protein, which, Ohsawa contends, is not suitable for human bodies, especially in the temperate zone. Since whole-grain brown rice and other grains are either 5 to 1 or close to that ratio of potassium to sodium, they are considered the staple food for human beings in this temperate climate, along with vegetables and other "natural" foods that are free of chemicals and pesticides and as close to their point of origin as possible.

Proponents of the diet and theory of macrobiotics claim that the proper balancing of food and its selection and preparation is the "way" to greater self-realization and happiness.

Magma

A thin paste or mixture; a precipitate tenaciously retaining liquid (water, alcohol) often removed only by forcible expression.

Magnesium

One of the metals found in alkaline earth, magnesium is a component of all vegetable and animal tissues. In the physiological sense, it enters into the composition of teeth and bones and is involved as a catalyst in metabolizing carbohydrates.

Magnesium deficiency is rare, but when it does occur, the signs include severe constipation, sleeplessness, nervousness, and extreme sensitivity to hot and cold.

When it is taken as a food supplement, magnesium acts as an antacid and a laxative. Small amounts of magnesium are found in a variety of foods, including citrus fruit, egg yolk, kelp, parsley, spinach, honey, and watercress.

Mammae

The mammae, or breasts, are two globular protrusions situated on each side of the breastbone. Each breast contains the mammary glands, which secrete antibodies, hormones, and, in women, convert nutrients to milk.

Manganese

A silver white metal which has properties similar to iron, manganese is known to affect the rate of release and use of nutrients by the body. It is used medicinally to improve appetite, as an antiseptic, and to stimulate the heart.

Manganese is found in natural form in almonds, liver, mint, parsley, unsalted olives, peanuts, potatoes, walnuts, and wheat germ.

Margarine

Margarine is a butter substitute which is made from seeds of cotton, sesame, olives, and soybeans. Because margarine is made entirely from vegetable fats, it contains no vitamin A, although some commercial processors of margarine add both vitamin A and vitamin D.

Massage

Rubbing and kneading the body in order to loosen up muscles and improve circulation. The term massage is derived from the Greek word *massein* or the French, *masser*—meaning "to knead." Passive manipulation of the soft tissues of the body is made directly on the skin in a methodical manner. The origin of the practice of massage has long since been lost in antiquity.

The kneading, stroking, and tapping of the body as a rule should be done toward the direction of the heart. This will cause a more rapid movement of the venous blood and allow it to be replaced by fresh arterial blood. Uses for massage include removal of wrinkles from the face and forehead, relief of strains, sprains, and muscular tension, and increase of circulation. A general massage requires from thirty-five to forty-five minutes, while ten to twenty minutes is sufficient for a local massage. The five fundamental manipulations of massage include effleurage (stroking), friction (rubbing), petrissage (kneading), tapotement (percussion), and vibration (shaking or trembling), sometimes accomplished with vibrators or other mechanical aids. (*See also Effleurage, Petrissage, Tapotement.*)

Materia Medica (Latin)

Literally, "medical material" is a treatise upon the materials, agents, or appliances used in medicine, including their names, sources (origins), habitats, families (natural organic order), physical characteristics, methods by which obtained, tests for purity and adulterations, constituents (composition), forms of administration (preparations), physiological actions (properties), uses (therapeutics, therapy), normal and lethal doses, antagonists, incompatibilities, synergists (organic and inorganic), and other important features.

Mead

A honey elixir used by the ancients for kidney disorders, rheumatism, and gout.

Meat

Meat is defined as the flesh of animals as used for food. Sometimes the term also includes fish and fowl. One should not eat meat in combination with large amounts of starchy foods. A good source of protein, meat also supplies a large amount of uric acid. It is easily digested if properly cooked, but should not be fried. Of all meats, pork is the least desirable. Lamb is least affected by enforced-growth chemicals and thus perhaps most preferable in terms of purity.

The harm in eating meat is often due to the manner of preparation. Those in good health will not experience any harm from eating meat when it is properly cooked and combined with other foods. There is an amino acid in meat which is necessary for human life.

An exclusive meat diet for the treatment of chronic diseases was used by physicians in England in the 1880s. They used the diet largely in the treatment of consumption. In taking the meat diet, round steak should be used, and all gristle and cartilage should be removed. It should then be ground finely, using little or no salt. This diet has been found valuable in the treatment of diabetes, Bright's disease, rheumatism, stomach troubles, constipation (particularly if used with celery), consumption, and other diseases.

Mechanotherapy

Mechanotherapy is the application of mechanical measures or the treatment of disease by means of manual manipulation. While massage is principally a passive form of exercise, mechanotherapy embraces all mechanical means including massage, Swedish movements, vibrations and other movements. The four kinds of movements recognized in mechanotherapy include (1) active movements, or those made entirely by the patient with her or his own strength; (2) passive movements, or those made entirely by the operator without any effort on the part of the patient; (3) active-passive or double-active movements (sometimes called duplicate active or eccentric movements), which are made by the operator and resisted by the patient.

While achieving much the same result as the massage, this method improves nerve function, digestion, and nutrition; increases muscular tone; raises body temperature; increases metabolism; breaks up adhesions and deposits in the joints, tendons, and so on; overcomes contraction of muscles and lengthens shrunken tissues; and prevents atrophy of muscles and improves circulation.

Mechanotherapy includes flexion and extension, lateral flexion, rotation, circumduction, abduction, adduction, pronation, supination, eversion, and inversion. Weak patients should not be treated too long, and the treatment should never be carried to the point of extreme fatigue. A slight fatigue is, however, to be expected. Mechanotherapy treatments should be used with extreme caution in such disorders as heart disease, high blood pressure, hemorrhage, spinal disease, acute inflammation, tumors, skin diseases, pregnancy, menstruation, abscesses, tubercular joints, and severe abdominal or pelvic pain.

Medicine Man or Shaman

The central figure in Indian healing, often called by the Asian term *shaman* by ethnologists, the medicine man is many things, including a healer, a sorcerer, a seer, an educator, and a priest. While at different times he is each of these, the way he represents himself depends upon the specialized need of the individual seeking his aid. Many practitioners used herbs, roots, and berries widely but claimed the cause of ailments was demons or evil spirits. Most medicine men or medicine women believe in the power of supernatural forces and have achieved results ranging from nothing to the miraculous. (See also *Indian Healing.*)

Medulla Oblongata

The expanded portion of the upper part of the spinal cord, it is pyramidal in form and is divided by the anterior and posterior median fissures. There are eight centers in the medulla: (1) cardiac center, which exerts an accelerator action over the heart's pulsations; (2) vasomotor center, which regulates the caliber of the blood vessels; (3) respiratory center, which coordinates muscles concerned with the production of the respiratory movements; (4) mastication center, which excites activity and coordinates the muscles of mastication; (5) deglutition center, which excites and coordinates the muscles involved in the transfer of food from the mouth to the stomach; (6) articulation center, which coordinates muscles necessary for production of articulate speech; (7) diabetic center, which stimulates the condition of glycosuria; and (8) salivary center, which stimulates the discharge of saliva.

Mel

A synonym for honey that also refers to medicines mixed with honey instead of syrup. The substance deposited in the honeycomb by the common honeybee, *Apis mellifica,* and a few other hymenopterous insects. It is emollient, nutritive, often laxative, and used as a vehicle for expectorant gargles and as a natural food sweetener.

Menthol

A substance obtained from oil of peppermint in the form of white crystals that give a cool taste or feeling, it is used often in salves and cough drops.

Mercury Quartz Lights

Mercury quartz lights generate artificial ultraviolet rays. It is known that the greatest effect of the sun is due to the ultraviolet rays. These therapeutic rays introduce certain chemical elements into the body that cause an increase of metabolism in all tissues. Such an action kills bacteria, increases oxidation, lowers pain, and modifies tissue.

The Alpine Sun Lamp and Kromayer Lamp produce ultraviolet rays that give maximum intensity for therapeutic procedures. The Alpine Sun Lamp is designed to irradiate large areas, while the Kromayer Lamp is adapted for treatment of localized areas such as the ear, eye, nose, throat, and other orifices.

Quartz-Light treatments are excellent for increasing hemoglobin and red blood cells. Its use stimulates the nervous system and the endocrine glands, raises vital resistance, and improves elimination.

In the beginning of treatment, the skin should be exposed to the light for about one minute. The duration of exposure should be gradually increased each day until treatment is continued for five to ten minutes or longer. If treatment is too long in the beginning, the skin will be burned instead of tanned. Fair-skinned persons and those with blond or red hair are inclined to react more quickly than darker persons. Quartz light is used therapeutically in every branch of medicine and surgery, as well as in natural practice.

Metaphysics

A philosophy which attempts to answer questions about what exists and can be known, metaphysics deals more in the abstract than in the material. The subject matter includes studies of God, numerology, astrology, ESP, tarot, palmistry, and so on.

Milk, Artificial (See *Milk, Modified*)

Milk, Composition

Goat's milk is a splendid diet and especially valuable in treating any pus-forming disease, as it contains blood salts to a marked degree. Goat's milk has more fluorine than any other food.

Composition of Goat's Milk

water	87.39%
protein	2.78
fat	3.84
sugar	4.25
ash	.81
lactic acid	.93

Goat's milk contains 315 calories per pint, or about 15 percent more than cow's milk, but is superior in chemical content.

Composition of Cow's Milk

water	87.0%
proteins	4.0
fats	4.0
sugar	4.3
salts	0.7

The mineral salts in cow's milk are made up of different mineral elements in varying quantities and occur, according to the quantity contained, in the following order: potassium, phosphorus, calcium, chlorine, sodium, magnesium, iron, sulphur, and silicon. If the patient does not respond to other forms of treatment, a milk diet can be tried using, when possible, raw, unpasteurized milk. The milk diet has remedied many complicated and obstinate diseases when all else has failed. Regular treatment may be given when patient is on the milk diet.

A substantial number of qualified and respected natural physicians believe that humans should consume only mother's milk as infants, and that large amounts of milk and dairy products in the adult diet are responsible for many disease conditions.

Milk, Drugs Excreted in

When drunk during lactation, the following substances, among others, are excreted in the milk: the oils of anise, cumin, dill, wormwood, and garlic, turpentine, the active principals of rhubarb, senna, scammony and castor oil, opium, iodine, indigo, antimony, arsenic bismuth, iron, lead, mercury, and zinc. Acids given to the mother cause griping in the child. Opium given to the mother may narcotize the child, and mercurials, in the same manner, may cause salivation.

Milk, Filtered

Milk may be satisfactorily filtered by placing it in a clean glass funnel lined with a piece of absorbent cotton about an inch thick and allowing the milk to percolate through it into the nursing bottle.

Milk, Modified

The modification of cow's milk consists of changing the proportions of different ingredients until they resemble as closely as possible those of mother's milk. To accomplish this, the proteins must be reduced by the addition of water; the sugar must be increased by adding cane sugar or milk sugar; the fats must be increased by using cream on account of dilution; an alkali such as sodium bicarbonate will be needed; and sterilization must be effected, preferably by the Pasteur method. (See *Infant Feeding.*)

Milk, Mother's

Colostrum is secreted for the first two or three days of lactation and differs quite markedly from the later milk; it is a deep yellow color and is not as sweet. Colostrum has a specific gravity of 1040 to 1060, coagulates into a solid mass when heated, is very rich in proteins and salts, and has a laxative effect. Looking through a microscope, besides fat globules, large numbers of granular bodies can be seen that are known as colostrum corpuscles. These gradually disappear from the milk by the end of a week to ten days. The first two days after parturition, the amount of milk secreted is very small, but after three to five days, there should be an abundant supply. Milk is continuously formed by the child suckling.

Milk flow may be influenced by prolonged nursing, age, severe fevers, pregnancy, belladonna and sometimes opium, iodides, bromides, salines, arsenic, mercury, salicylates, and various nervous impressions. Nitrogenous foods increase fats and proteins. A vegetable diet diminishes fats and proteins. A very meager diet diminishes the fats and may either increase or diminish proteins. An excessively rich diet increases both fats and proteins. Liquids increase the quantity. Alcoholic drinks or malt extracts increase the quantity, as well as fats and usually proteins. Massage of the breasts is one of the most efficient means of stimulating the milk supply.

An easy clinical test of the milk is as follows: too high specific gravity shows excess of proteins, too low specific gravity, excess of fats. The sugar and salts are practically constant. To ascertain the percentage of fats, take a cylinder holding 10 cubic centimeters graduated to 100 parts. Fill to the 100 mark with the milk and allow the cream to rise for twenty-four hours. The cream bears a relation of 5 to 3 of the fat, so if the reading on the cylinder shows 7 of cream, the fats would equal three-fifths of that, or 4.2 percent. The following table gives the average percentage of the different ingredients in cow's milk and mother's milk:

	Cow's Milk	*Mother's Milk*
fats	4.00%	4.00%
sugar	4.30	7.00
protein	4.00	1.50
salts	0.70	0.20
water	87.00	87.30
specific gravity	1029	1031
reaction	acid	alkaline
	(not sterile)	(sterile)

Milk, Pasteurized

Milk is pasteurized by heating it to a temperature of 167° F for 20 minutes. This process has been shown to be sufficient to destroy the germs (but not their spores) most commonly found in milk. Milk thus treated will keep two or three hours in a room at ordinary temperature and in a refrigerator for about a week.

Milk, Peptonized

Peptonized milk (or other predigested food) is used when the natural digestive powers are enfeebled or suspended. The following is a simple method for peptonizing milk: in a clean glass jar containing 4 ounces of cold distilled or boiled water, dissolve 15 grains of bicarbonate of sodium and 5 grams of pancreatin (*extractum pancreatis*). Add 12 ounces of milk. Set the jar in a vessel of water at a temperature of 106 to 115° F for 5 to 20 minutes to partially peptonize, and for 2 hours to completely digest or peptonize. (See *Peptonized Food.*)

Milk, Sterilized

Sterilized milk is that in which the germs have been destroyed by heat. The common method of sterilizing is to place the milk in jars, which are then exposed to the action of steam for an hour and a half. The quality of the milk is altered by this method, and it should be used only when other procedures such as pasteurizing are impossible.

Minerals

Substances that have been formed in the earth by nature, especially inorganic ones such as iron, sodium, and magnesium. Many of these minerals are essential to good health and are sold as health aids.

Mineral Salts (Daily Requirements)

U.S. Recommended Daily Allowances (RDA) from the Food and Drug Administration standards for nutrition labeling of foods,* based on the 1968 RDA.

	Adults and Children over 4	*Infants and Children under 4*
calcium	1 gram	0.8 grams
iron	18 milligrams	10 milligrams
phosphorus	1 gram	0.8 grams
iodine	150 micrograms	70 micrograms
magnesium	400 milligrams	200 milligrams
zinc	15 milligrams	8 milligrams
copper	2 milligrams	1 milligram

*No commercially produced food provides more than 150 percent of the RDA. Amounts in excess of this are classified as drugs.

Mineral Springs

Widely sought out throughout the United States and Europe, the waters of mineral springs have brought relief to thousands of persons suffering from chronic disorders. Hundreds of cures have reportedly been effected by drinking and bathing in these waters. The benefit is derived not so much from the mineral content of the water as it is from the fact that the patient drinks large quantities of the water and bathes in it daily for extended periods. The mineral waters are usually very warm, and the constant bathing and drinking keep the pores of the skin open so the poisons and morbid matter from the system can be eliminated. Drinking copious quantities of water keeps the bowels and kidneys active, and frequent bathing keeps the pores in the skin open, thus stimulating the three principal channels for eliminating waste material from the body. As retention of waste matter in the system is an underlying cause of the majority of chronic disorders, one can readily understand why people receive so much benefit from stays at such mineral springs.

An excellent substitute for many mineral springs can be readily made by dissolving a cup of Epsom Salts and a tablespoon of common salt in a tub half-full of water (or 21 gallons). Some practitioners advise a cup of Epsom Salts and Glauber's salt or sodium sulfate (3 parts to 2 parts), in the same amount of water. The patient can then achieve the benefit of the mineral water by drinking this water as well as frequently bathing in it.

Mint (See *Peppermint, Spearmint*)

Miracle Cures

In this modern day, miracle cures seem beyond belief for many. Still, a stream of injured, blind, and disabled people, all suffering, continues to flock to places such as Lourdes and Padua—and many come away cured.

The word *miracle* is derived from the Latin *miraculum,* meaning a wonderful occurrence. A miracle is a visible and extraordinary event produced *in* nature but not *by* nature. It is above the powers of all natural agencies and is brought about by the intervention of the divine powers of God, either through His beloved devotees or directly. It always excites wonder, striking an awesome contrast between itself and the ordinary natural event. Being a deviation from the natural law, it is an anomaly, an aberration, an exception.

Critics use modern science as the weapon to destroy belief in miracles. But science limited by natural law has always proved to be a poor argument against supernatural or divine powers. We must distinguish between *science* and *scientists.* Some scientists repeat the formula that since the laws of nature are constant and uniform in their operation, miracles are a contradiction of this rule. But a miracle is an exception to the rule and therefore proves the rule. So far as natural order is concerned, the laws of nature are certainly uniform, but once the supernatural or divine order is admitted, the possibility of its interfering with the natural order must also be admitted. Hence science is a poor argument to discard miracles which have been testified to by many eminent scientists, physiologists, and medical people of our age.

Moeller System

Dr. Siegfried Moeller used the fast in his practice, and himself fasted several times up to twenty-five days. To Moeller, fasting was an excellent means to "regain possession of mind and body faculties." Moeller fasted often and gladly, not only to overcome minor body discomforts but mainly to compensate for vacations he could not afford to take. An as overworked physician in a sanatorium, his "frequent vacations" consisted of taking short fasts of from six to ten days. By this method, Moeller claimed, he could maintain his overexertions in his work despite an inherited weak constitution.

Morse Wave Generator

A combination of sine-wave and galvanic-current mechanisms, the Morse Wave Generator produces a current of much higher frequency than sinusoidal current and is the best device to produce involuntary exercise of muscular tissues. (See *Electrotherapy*.)

Moxibustion

A form of therapy used in the Far East, moxibustion is a token form of burning, often effected with leaf down from wormwood or sunflower pith, although cotton wool has been used occasionally. The principles of application are nearly identical to those of acupuncture. There is comparatively little reliable literature on this art, and efforts to trace any authoritative body such as exists for many other forms of healing have met with failure. It is reported to be as efficacious as acupuncture.

Mucilages

Saturated aqueous adhesive liquids of gum or starch.

Mucusless Diet Healing System

This extension of dietetics is based on an attempt to free the mucous membranes of all impurities. The mucous membranes are, broadly speaking, the inside continuation of the skin of the body. This thin lining covers the parts of the body which have any access to the outside of the body, such as the lungs, the respiratory system, the mouth and digestive system, and all parts connected with eating and drinking. It consists of several layers of tiny glands, which produce a liquid secretion to keep the top layer mobile and fluid. This protects the surface from being injured by irritating substances and hot foods. For people with a bad cold or constipation, hot food or drinks always produce an intensification of the stuffiness and discomfort that are symptomatic of their condition. Substances such as apple-cider vinegar, orange juice, lemon and grapefruit juice (and these fruits eaten whole) do much to relieve symptoms, toning up the membranes. One of the well-known practitioners of the mucusless system was Arnold Ehret (1866–1922), who set forth his practice in *Muscusless Diet Healing System* (Beaumont, Calif.: Ehret Publishing Co., 1922).

Mud Baths

These are of value in disorders of an inflammatory nature. To give a mud bath, clay or peat earth is moistened and worked into a soft mass. Several pails of the mud are spread upon a large piece of canvas, and the patient is placed upon this. More mud is spread upon the body until it is well covered. The canvas is then wrapped around the body and the patient allowed to remain in the mud for from forty-five minutes to one hour. The patient is then given a shower and dried. The mud should be heated to a temperature of 98 to 100°F. As a local application, mud is of value in cases of boils, poisonous bites, and sores.

Mugwort *(Artemisia vulgaris)*

This plant grows wild in the United States. The leaves are the medicinal part, which the American Indians used for treatment of colds, colic, bronchitis, rheumatism, and fever. It is a safe remedy for suppressed menstruation and effective for various female complaints when combined with marigold.

Mugwort is also important in the treatment of kidney and bladder inflammations and related ailments such as gout, sciatica, and water retention. The herb has even been used as an antidote to opium. Dosage is 1 teaspoonful to 1 cup of boiling water steeped for 20 minutes, taken in 4 ounce amounts.

Mullein *(Verbascum thapsus)*

Native to Europe, North Africa, and central and western Asia, the medicinal portions of mullein are the leaves, flowers, and root. Some of its many uses include treatment of coughs, colds, and pectoral complaints including hemorrhages of the lungs, shortness of breath, and pulmonary illness. Mullein has been considered an effective treatment for hemorrhoids for hundreds of years and is still used for this, both internally and as a fomentation. Dosage is 1 teaspoon of the leaves or flowers to 1 cup of boiling water. Dosage of the tincture is 15 to 40 drops in warm water every two to four hours.

Mullein was used in Germany as a remedy for deafness resulting from dried earwax, soft earwax, or insufficient earwax. A fomentation of leaves in hot vinegar forms an excellent local application for inflamed piles, ulcers, tumors, mumps, acute inflammation of the tonsils, malignant sore throat, dropsy of the joints, sciatica, spinal tenderness, and so on. A mixture of simmered leaves can also be inhaled through a teapot spout for many of the aforementioned conditions.

Mulls

Hard ointments (suet- and lard-based) spread on soft muslin or "mull" similar to plasters.

Muscle Test (See *Kinesiology*)

Mushrooms

Small, fleshy fungi that grow very fast, with the stalk topped with caps in various shapes. Some kinds may be eaten and are relished by many gourmets. Others of the same family are poisonous and are called toadstools. While the mushroom is known to be a fine source of nourishment, it is important to insure proper identification to avoid gathering a poisonous variety in the wild.

Musk

Musk comes from the dried secretions of the preputial gland of the muskdeer of Tibet and has a marked odor. It is a diffusible stimulant, supportive to the heart, an antispasmodic and a nerve sedative, and is used in enemas in the crises of low fevers, in a dosage of up to 6 grams. It is not to be employed except to carry a patient past a crisis. (See also *Sumbul.*)

Mustard *(Jinapis nigra)*

The seed of this herb is principally used for culinary purposes, for which it is ground into a very fine powder and mixed with warm water. It is very pungent and of a hot nature, but it is volatile and will not hold heat long enough to do much for internal heat retention. It is good for creating an appetite and assisting the digestion; given sweetened in hot water, it will remove pain in the bowels and stomach. It is frequently used for the treatment of rheumatism, both internally and externally. A mustard plaster is a valuable counterirritant in the treatment of pain in the abdomen or chest. It should be made by mixing mustard flour in varying proportions with ordinary flour, moistened with warm vinegar or water. Half mustard and half wheat flour will suffice if the skin is tender, but for children, one-fourth mustard is strong enough. The addition of a raw egg to the mixture tends to retard excess burning of the skin. To make the plaster, place a piece of heavy muslin on a newspaper, over which smear the mustard mass. On top of this, place a thin piece of muslin to prevent adhesions to the skin and modify the irritant effect. The edges of the newspaper may be folded to resemble a picture frame and the plaster placed within this, giving it support. Mustard burns are peculiar in their slowness to heal and in the fact that they are tender and reddened for days. When the burning is excessive, a piece of lint soaked in lime water and olive oil may be used to give relief. Vaseline can also be spread over the burned area.

Myrrh *(Commiphora molmol)*

A gum resin obtained from the *Commiphora molmol,* a tree of Arabia, myrrh is a dark brownish-red, and has an agreeable aromatic odor and a bitter acrid taste. In medicinal amounts, it is a stimulant to the circulation and to the uterine and bronchial mucous membranes. It is used locally in ulcerative stomatitus, ptyalism, and acute pharyngitis; internally, in combination with other herbs for chronic bronchitis and functional amenorrhea. The average dosage is 8 grams.

Naprapathy

The science of naprapathy was founded by Oakley Smith in 1905 and continued to develop under his direction at his college and clinic in Chicago, Illinois, until his death in 1970 at the age of ninety.

Naprapathic treatment consists of charted ligamentous manipulation of the spine and its supporting muscles. The purpose of the treatment is to stretch shrunken ligamentous tissue (called ligatite) and return blood and nerve flow to a normal and balanced condition.

Some naprapathic practitioners also employ the use of light, heat, sound, dietetics, food supplements, and other hygienic measures to assist in correcting the ligatites. The practice of naprapathy is not presently licensed in any state, although there are many practitioners of this art in Chicago, most having been graduated from the National College of Naprapathy there. The only other functioning college of naprapathy is located in Phoenix, Arizona.

Natural Childbirth

The process of birthing new life is by and large natural in and of itself, and the term used here denotes the creation of an environment in harmony with the sensitive moment of spiritual release which may often be part of the actual moments of birth. This is in contrast to the ordinary hospital birth, which often is a cold and impersonal experience for the mother and newborn infant.

Those who desire "natural childbirth," according to one meaning of the term, may elect to supervise the birth itself, sometimes with the assistance of a professional or lay midwife or a medical doctor who has agreed to supervise a home birth; or the father or other close relative may deliver the child without any help.

A second meaning of the term refers to those who undergo a period of physical and psychological training prior to the birth, usually for about six weeks, during which the mother and father learn much about the physiological events which will attend the birth and practice breathing patterns to assist the birth process. The Lamaze Method is one such system which is widely available, with classes offered through many hospitals, local midwife groups, or other health groups. The intent of such classes is to build closeness between parents and child, to allay fears and anxiety about the birth, and, by physical instructions, to endeavor to allow the mother to avoid as much as possible the use of drugs during delivery. Many hospitals, no doubt responding to the demands of the general public, have converted the ordinarily stark labor and delivery rooms into warm, "homey" environments, which reflect as much as possible a desire to reduce the sense of childbirth being a "disease" process.

Natural Food

In the 1970s in the United States, with the proliferation of modalities of improving the general state of health, a considerable expansion of sales of products described as "natural," "organic," or "health" foods occurred. However, there is no specific definition of exactly what constitutes a "natural" food, although there is general agreement that it means, at the minimum, foods that have been grown from uncontaminated seeds, in organic soil, with no chemical fertilizers or pesticides employed. Nonetheless, many commercial food processors still advertise their products as both natural and organic, when chemical tests have shown that undesirable components such as refined sugar are present.

To arrive at an acceptable definition of natural food substances, the underlying notion that the chemical composition of blood and lymph depends upon the chemical composition of food and drink, and upon the normal or abnormal condition of the digestive organs, must be accepted. The purer the food and drink, the less it contains of morbid matter and the more it contains those nutrients necessary for building and repair of tissue and for neutralizing chemical food additives and toxic products of digestion.

The system of dietetics of the nature-cure practitioners who founded naturopathy in this country in the early 1900s is based upon the composition of pure, raw cow's milk, which is considered the most complete natural food combination in nature. This notion has been challenged to some degree in the past few years by adherents of other food systems, such as those of the macrobiotic way, who claim that diets or food substances which can qualify as "natural" should conform as closely as possible in chemical composition to that of milk or red, arterial blood.

At the time of the writing of this book, there are efforts underway by several consumer groups, natural physicians, and others to provide a legal definition of what constitutes a natural, organic food substance, and only those foods or products meeting such criteria would be allowed to be advertised as "natural." Until such a legal definition is successfully constructed and put into practice, much debate over the nature of natural foods will be likely to continue. (See *Organic Food.*)

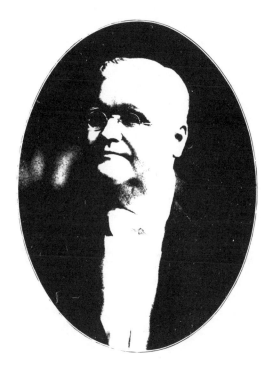

Henry Lindlahr, an early twentieth century medical doctor considered by many to be the father of nature cure in America, founded his system upon the simple statement, "Nature's remedies are the best."

Nature Cure

Nature cure is the name coined by a medical physician, Henry Lindlahr, who, at the turn of the twentieth century, was one of the pioneers of natural therapeutics in the United States. He set forth several important principles which seem to have withstood the test of time and are succinct in reviewing the essentials of natural-cure philosophy.

According to Lindlahr, nature cure is a system of building the health of the human body in harmony with the constructive principle in nature of the physical, mental, and moral planes of being. The constructive principle is understood to mean all things which build up, improve, and repair. Disease is seen to be an inharmonious or abnormal vibration of the elements and forces composing the human entity, and is primarily caused by violation of "natural laws." The effects of violation of these laws include lowered vitality, abnormal composition of blood and lymph, and accumulation of morbid materials, waste matter, and poisons—all of which promote destruction of healthy tissues.

While there are many dozens of treatment modalities employed in the practice of nature cure, the basic ideals of the treatments are: (1) to establish normal surroundings and natural habits of life; (2) to economize the natural life force; (3) to build up the blood by supplying correct nutrients in proper proportions; (4) to promote elimination of waste materials and toxins without damaging the function of eliminative organs; (5) to correct mechanical lesions; and (6) to arouse in people the highest possible degree of consciousness of personal responsibility, in the form of intelligent individual effort and self-help.

Many practitioners adhere to the nature-cure system in philosophy and practice, including chiropractors, naturopaths, naprapaths, herbalists, osteopaths, some medical physicians, and all the allied health practices such as yoga, spiritual counseling, massage, rolfing, and related systems of restoring the body to optimum health levels. (See also *Naturopathy.*)

Naturopathy

The term *naturopathy* was coined in the United States by Dr. Bennedict Lust, M.D., to mean the inclusion of all forms of health care that strengthen and cleanse the body so as to prevent disease and return the body to a condition of stasis.

The history of medicine since its recorded origins abounds in references to and use of natural means of maintaining or returning the body to health. The earliest physicians, who were often either religious persons or spiritually advanced as a requirement of their training, used herbs and other natural therapies, including diets and fasting, exercise, massage, heat and cold therapeutics, and many other modalities.

In the late 1800s and early 1900s, many American medical doctors visited Europe and learned the "nature cure" methods from the famous clinics of that time. Dr. W. K. Kellogg, of Rice Krispies fame, was in fact a medical doctor who practiced nature-cure methods and operated a nature-cure sanitarium at Battle Creek, Michigan (he developed not only a line of health food cereals but also invented peanut butter).

While Dr. Lust and many others were practicing and advancing the nature-cure concept in the United States, naturopathy as a science flourished in a rather unscientific manner until the publication in 1951 of *Standardized Naturopathy,* by Dr. Paul Wendel (Wendel: Brooklyn, 1951). This book provided, for the first time, an exhaustive listing and organization of the methods which fall within the confines of "naturopathic treatment," comprising nearly three hundred different modalities. What they have in common is that they employ no chemical drugs and perform no major surgery.

When naturopathy seemed about to be organized into a full-fledged healing science, the spectacular scientific advances of allopathic medicine eclipsed the nature healers, who were portrayed as "old-fashioned." In nearly every state and part of the country, they were either hounded out of practice or laws were enacted specifically to prevent them from practicing. Still, some practitioners conducted their healing secretly or under the cover of some legally recognized but related modality, such as massage or dietary therapy.

With the resurgence of interest in holistic medicine in the late 1960s, naturopathy also experienced a renewal, and today nearly half the states legally recognize naturopathy as a healing profession. However, the requirements for licensing are difficult to satisfy and vary widely by state. Basically there are three conditions of the law at present in regard to naturopathy: some states do not legalize it but allow it; some states regulate the practice by statute; and other states specifically prohibit its practice by statute.

One reason for naturopathy's slow growth is a lack of schools and facilities for training practitioners, although since 1975, several new schools have instituted programs (some, however, have inadequate library and laboratory facilities). Some European naturopathic colleges of high caliber exist, but acceptance of credits earned abroad is at present not allowed by most United States licensing boards. The designation of N.D. (Doctor of Naturopathy) signifies one who has completed training in a formal program of naturopathy. Information on degree programs in naturopathy in the United States is available from the National College of Naturopathic Medicine, Room 413, 510 SW Third Avenue, Portland, Oregon 97204. (See also *Nature Cure.*)

Nauheim Bath

Also known as the *Schott Treatment,* these baths are popular primarily in Germany, being employed in cases of cardiac diseases, kidney disorders, rheumatism, and many nervous conditions, including sexual malfunctions in men and women.

At European spas which offer this treatment, a specially prepared artifical salt compound is used The following formula is often used as a substitute:

> 1½ pounds table salt
> 7 ounces bicarbonate of soda
> 10½ ounces muriatic acid

The soda and salt are dissolved in approximately 12 gallons of water, and the muriatic acid mixed into 1½ pints of pure water. The diluted muriatic acid is put into a syringe and placed above a tub full of water in which the patient is seated. The diluted acid is then allowed to flow into the bottom of the tub, producing small bubbles of effervescence. The water temperature is adjusted to 95° F, and the bath lasts about 8 minutes. The baths are repeated every third day for a total of about a dozen treatments, with the water temperature being gradually lowered in increments of 1 degree per bath.

As this treatment involves the use of a highly caustic and dangerous acid, it is *absolutely not* recommended for self-administration but should be undertaken only under the advice and direct supervision of a licensed doctor.

Nerve Cells

The nerve cell is the individual unit of the nervous system. Nourishment is received from the arterioles and lymphatics, and by-products are drained away by venules. Each nerve cell has two functions, the *axis cylinder process* and the *protoplasmic process*. The cell itself, along with the two processes, is known as a *neuron*. The axis cylinder process conveys impulses away from the cells, and the protoplasmic process directs current into the cells.

The brain, spinal cord, and various nerve ganglia throughout the body are examples of nerve-cell complexes.

Neuropractic

A system of specific nerve pressure developed by a chiropractic doctor, M. O. Garten. He inadvertently discovered that pain could be relieved by applying pressure to specific nerve centers and nerve pathways. The treatment, concentrated usually on the feet, consists of steady pressure to the point of pain, followed by light massage. The pressure applications and manipulations may have some relation to acupuncture meridians, but Dr. Garten systematized his findings into a textbook for manipulative professions. At present, neuropractics is not taught in formal schools in the United States, nor is it licensed by any official body.

Nicolini Method

This method was initiated by Dr. Juan Nicolini Mena, a Mexican, who died in 1956. His theory holds that cancer is primarily due to an acid-base imbalance in the cells, which can be detected by the Methylene Blue Test which is used to discover precipitates of organic and mineral salts, by-products of abnormal acid-base balance.

The method of treatment is first to determine the chemical components of the blood, after which several kinds of prepared "Nicolini sera" are given by injection. These medications are progressively numbered from one to ten, depending upon their pH value. Another physician, Dr. Xavier Farias, wrote a monograph titled "Theory and Method of the Nicolini Method," and also developed his own injectable sera in addition to those developed by Nicolini.

Niehans Cellular Therapy

Paul Niehans was born in Berne, Switzerland, in 1887. He was a nephew of Wilhelm II, emperor of Germany, and was exhaustively educated at the leading institutions of his day, receiving doctorate degrees in theology, science, medicine, and medical philosophy.

He began research into cellular biology with Alexis Carrel in Paris before World War I and later was appointed by Pope Pius XII to the Pontifical Academy of Sciences of Rome. Dr. Niehans discovered his cellular treatment in 1931 and claimed to have successfully treated more than thirty thousand patients with it during his lifetime.

Cellular therapeutics is a method of regenerating the trillions of cells of the body by means of making available to them cells from animal embryos and young animals. Fresh tissue cells are injected by hypodermic needle into the upper, outer quadrant of the buttocks.

Practically all forms of disease have been reported to respond to cellular therapy, with the specific cellular material to be used being at the discretion of the physician. The success of the treatment is tied to successful diagnosis of the particular organ affected with degeneration; proper determination of vitamin, mineral, and cell-salt deficiency; and the level of various chemicals and toxins in the body.

Owing to a Food and Drug Administration ban on importation of the raw cellular materials, there are at present few practitioners of this form of therapy in the United States. Additional information on clinics and physicians employing this treatment in other parts of the world may be obtained from The International Association of Cancer Victors and Friends (IACVF). (See *Nontoxic Therapies.*)

Dr. Niehan's book, *Introduction to Cellular Therapy,* was published in 1960 by Pageant Books, Cooper Square Publishers, 59 Fourth Avenue, New York, New York.

Nontoxic Therapies

This term has entered the English language to describe therapies used primarily to treat cancer by nonsurgical, nonchemical means. However, many of the therapies and treatments developed in the past fifty years do involve ingestion of substances which may be as toxic as orthodox medical treatments. Nontoxic therapies now number nearly a hundred, although few of them are readily available in the United States. Information on all the nontoxic therapies, along with information on practitioners in various parts of the world, is available from International Association of Cancer Victors and Friends, 7740 West Manchester Avenue, Suite 110, Playa Del Ray, California, 90291.

The clinic of Hans Nieper, M.D., located at 21 Sudanstrasse 3000, Hanover, Germany, has the reputation for being the finest facility in the world for treatment of cancer. All forms of therapy, orthodox and nontoxic, are offered; they are prescribed on an individual basis by medical doctors.

In the Western hemisphere, a clinic similar in approach to the one in Germany is operated by Dr. Marco Brown, Director of the Fairfield Medical Center; P.O. Box 1296; Montego Bay, Jamaica, West Indies.

(See also: *Blass Oxygen Therapy, Electrolyte Rejuvenation Program, Enderlein Therapy, Gerson Therapy, Grape Diet , Hydrochloric Acid Therapy, Glyoxylide, Krebiozen and Carcalon, Laetrile, Macrobiotics, Niehans Cellular Therapy, Nicolini Method.*)

Nose

The nose is divided into the external parts, consisting of skin, cartilage, and bone; and the internal parts, made up of nasal fossae which connect with the pharynx.

The nose constantly secretes a thick mucus, which catches foreign particles as they come into the nasal cavity. It also slightly warms the air before it is passed into the lungs.

In the upper portion of the nasal cavity are endings of the olfactory nerves, which control the sense of smell.

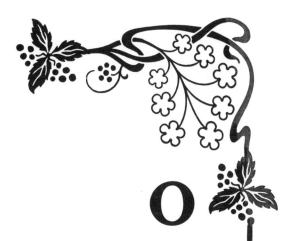

Oak *(Quercus)*

A large tree with hard wood and nuts called acorns. Many American Indian tribes make a bitter tea from the crushed meat of the acorn, which is believed to have a strengthening and immunizing value. The bark of the white oak variety *(Quercus alba)* contains tannic acid, and its infusion is used as an astringent application in the treatment of leucorrhea, vaginitis, prolapsus ani, hemorrhoids, and so on.

Oak (Poison)

A poisonous shrub related to poison ivy. The plant has leaves growing three in a cluster and is most dangerous in the fall, when the leaves turn red. Contact results in a rash developing into a blistering, runny mass, which spreads quickly. It can be transferred from touch, clothing, wind, and smoke. Treatment includes calamine lotion and various herbs.

Obstetrics

The branch of medicine dealing with the care of women who are giving birth. The practitioner's care usually begins soon after conception and continues through delivery of the newborn. (See *Natural Childbirth.*)

Occupational Therapy

A highly specialized form of therapy designed to prepare the handicapped, whatever their potential may be, for an occupation or employment in the effort to help them become as self-sustaining as possible.

Oils

Liquid active constituents, obtained by distillation or expression.

Ointments

Soft or solid fatty preparations, for external use, liquefying when rubbed upon the skin, and containing medicine in a basis of petrolatum, wool fat, prepared suet, expressed oil of almond, wax, spermacetti, paraffin, etc. *Salve* and *paste* are names often applied by lay people to healing ointments.

Oleates

Solutions of medicines (alkaloids or metallic salts) in oleic acid.

Oleoresins

Natural solutions of resin in volatile oils, extracted by ether, acetone, or alcohol.

Opium Poppy *(Papaver somnifermum)*

The inspissated juice of unripe capsules of the *Papaver somnifermum*, or opium poppy. It contains several alkaloids, the principals of which are morphine and codeine. Opium is used to relieve pain from any cause except acute inflammation of the brain, to produce sleep, to allay irritation, to check excessive secretion, and to support the system in low fevers and adynamic conditions when sufficient food cannot be retained. It causes slowing of the respiration and pulse, contracting of the pupils, diaphoresis, constipation, and, on rare occasions, nausea, vomiting, headache, erythema, wakefulness, delirium, and convulsions. When taken in toxic doses, these effects are exaggerated and death can result from paralysis of the respiratory center.

Children withstand opium badly, and its proportionate dosage should be much smaller than that of other agents. When given to a nursing mother, opium will affect the child. Poisoning by opium will require the immediate evacuation of the stomach by emetics or by a stomach tube.

Organic Food

Food grown without the use of chemical fertilizers, additive, insecticides, or sprays. Organic fruits and vegetables are grown with natural fertilizer only and without the use of chemical sprays. Organic meats are derived from animals given no chemical stimulants to induce growth or tenderness. (See *Natural Food.*)

Orificial (Bloodless) Surgery (See *Psychic Surgery*)

Orthopathy

Any way of restoring health by correcting the intake of foods and other substances into the body. Coming from the Greek root ortho-, meaning to "correct," it is a general term which covers many of the specific therapies described in this book.

Osteopathy

The system of healing known as osteopathy was founded by Andrew Still (1828–1917). He found that he could diagnose conditions by touching areas of the body in order to judge the speed of heat and quality of blood palpitating beneath those areas. It is not too different from the healing system known as radiesthesia and bears some relationship to the theory of vital force channels referred to by adherents of acupuncture.

Still's researches produced some amazing results. He pointed out that many illnesses have a relationship to disorders of the spine and could be reversed by manipulating the joints back into correct alignment, as well as that sicknesses such as erysipelas and many types of respiratory ailments could be healed by this method. The basis of Still's research emphasized the way in which illness can be related to a condition of the whole body and is not an isolated outbreak in just one organ or area.

The advantages of Still's methods are that cures can be virtually instantaneous. When the cause of the affliction is removed, the conditions set up by that cause disappear quickly. Practitioners of osteopathy, however, are aware of certain limits, such as that vitamin and mineral-salt deficiencies are often behind the loss of muscular tone and the consequent misalignment of the skeletal structure. Osteopathy offers bloodless surgery in the form of manipulation,

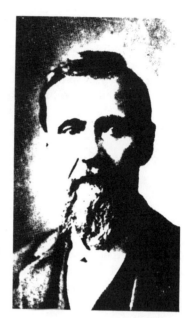

Andrew Still (1828-1917), founder of osteopathy.

which often cures chronic conditions. Certain arthritic conditions such as slipped discs, asthmatic-bronchitic conditions that may be due to lesions of the spine behind the shoulder blades, muscular atrophy, the Parkinson syndrome, pneumonia, and most forms of dislocation known have all yielded to the touch of osteopaths.

Modern osteopaths work with X-rays to examine the position of the joints, paying special attention to spinal lesions, which, it is generally known, influence the entire body by exerting pressure on the nervous system and blood vessels. Osteopaths refer to the lymph as the fluids of life and believe that unless the lymphatic system, as well as the circulation of the blood, is working properly, the patient will suffer from a buildup of artificial chemicals, toxic substances, and chlorinated hydrocarbons of mercury.

Still was strongly opposed to alcoholic drink and to any substances which induced autointoxication into the body.

Oxygen

A colorless, odorless, tasteless gas composing one-fifth of the atmosphere, eight-ninths of water, three-fourths of organized bodies, and about one-half of the crust of the globe. It is inhaled as a therapeutic agent in diseases of the respiratory organs and blood. It is essential to respiration; its combination with the tissues yields heat and other energy. It exists also in an allotropic form known as ozone.

Oxygen Therapy (See *Blass Oxygen Therapy*)

Oxymel

A preparation used in medieval times, believed to be a mixture of honey, water, and vinegar. It was used as a remedy for gout and sciatica. Also as a mixture of honey, sea water, rain water, and vinegar, it was used in ancient times for rheumatic conditions.

Ozone

An allotropic form of oxygen, its molecule having the structure of O_3. It is an active oxidizing agent, possessing bleaching and antiseptic properties. Ozone is generated by high-frequency current. Ozone generators are manufactured for hooking up to high-frequency generators. The ozone is collected so that it can be inhaled, after it is passed through special oils which purify the ozone, removing objectionable nitrous and nitric oxides.

Ozone is a concentrated form of oxygen that is soothing to tissues. It causes an increase in oxygen and the number of red blood cells in the body. It purifies the blood, disinfects, deodorizes, and is a powerful antiseptic. Diseases which have responded to ozone treatment are asthma, catarrh, colds, coughs, hay fever, bronchitis, pneumonia, and all diseases of the respiratory tract. (See also *Violet Ray*.)

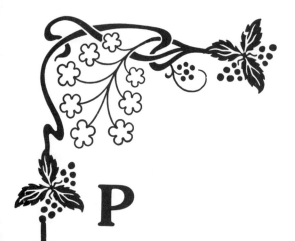

P

P Vitamin

There is little argument among proponents of vitamin therapy that vitamin P is essential, although little is known at present regarding its properties or distribution. In fact, some researchers even claim that substances of the P group are no longer considered vitamins.

It appears, however, to be abundant in lemon juice and is probably present in other citrus juices. Until the uncertainty regarding vitamin P is removed, it is preferable, whenever possible, to use the natural antiscorbutic foods—citrus and tomato juices and vegetables. However, if these fruits and vegetables are unavailable, pure synthetic vitamin C is a good substitute.

Vitamin P is believed to tone up arterial and capillary systems throughout the body and to prevent high blood pressure. Found sometimes in other fruits, it is also called rutin or bioflavonida. Grapes and rose hips also contain traces of this vitamin.

Pack (Cold, Hot, Half, and Wet)

A pack may be used to reduce temperature or to produce sweating. (See *Hot Packs.*)

A cold pack is a blanket wrung out of cold water and wrapped about the body. A half-pack is limited to the trunk of the body. A hot pack is a blanket wrung out of hot water and wrapped about the body. A wet pack is a blanket wrung out of warm or cold water and wrapped about the whole body, or only a part of it, and surrounded by dry blankets.

Palate

The palate forms the roof of the mouth. It consists of the hard part in the front and the soft portion in the back. The hard palate is formed by a part of

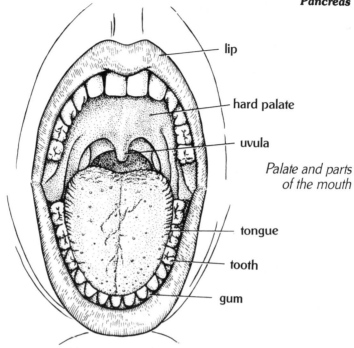

lip

hard palate

uvula

*Palate and parts
of the mouth*

tongue

tooth

gum

the maxilla and the horizontal plate of the palate bone. It is covered with a mucous membrane, which is closely adherent to the periosteum and forms along the median line a linear ridge. The soft palate is movable, suspended from the posterior border of the hard palate, and forms an incomplete septum between the mouth and pharynx. It consists of a fold of mucous membrane, enclosing muscular fibers.

Palmistry

The practice of attempting to reveal one's future by studying the lines of the hand. Those who employ palmistry use it as a means of opening up and clearing perceptions of reality. It teaches them how to look at life from all angles and thus, with the knowledge gained, to take control of the energies of life and the environment. The study falls into the class of the esoteric or metaphysical and is believed by some to be essential to complete understanding of the self and its relation to life.

Pancreas

The pancreas is a compound gland approximately 5½ inches broad, situated transversely across the posterior of the abdomen behind the stomach and in

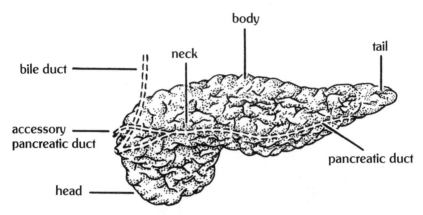

front of the first lumbar vertebra. The pancreas communicates with the large intestine by means of the duct of Wirsung. This duct commences at the tail and runs transversely through the body of the gland. As it approaches the head of the gland, it gradually increases in size until it measures about two or three millimeters in diameter. It then curves downward and forward and opens into the duodenum. On its course through the gland, the duct receives branches which enter it nearly at right angles. Pancreatic juice is transparent, colorless, strongly alkaline, and viscid, and has a specific gravity of 1.02. It is one of the most important of the digestive fluids, as it exerts a transforming influence upon all classes of alimentary principles and has been shown to contain at least three enzymes.

Pancreatin

A mixture of the enzymes of the pancreas, it is also the commercial extract of the pancreas. Added to fats, milk, soups, or gruels, the dosage is 8 grains.

Papain

A proteolytic ferment obtained from papaw milk, which is the juice of *Carica papaya,* a tree native to South America. It has the digestive properties of pepsin but is far more active.

Parabenzoquinone (PBQ)

An oxidation agent consisting of 6 parts per million of parabenzoquinone in distilled water. It is said to have value in treating certain diseases, including allergies, viral and bacterial colds, and cancer.

Parathyroids

Small glands, usually four in number, located close to or on the thyroid gland. The *superior* parathyroids are situated internally—on the posterior surface in close relation to, and frequently imbedded in, the thyroid; the *inferior* parathyroids are situated adjacent to the thyroid.

Peach Meats

The meats within the peach pit or stone have long been used as medicine and are of great value in strengthening the stomach and bowel and restoring the digestion. Made into a cordial with other ingredients, peach meat is one of the best remedies to aid the recovery of the natural tone of the stomach after prolonged illness. It is also excellent for the restoration of weak patients, particularly following dysentery. A tea made of the leaves of the peach tree is an excellent remedy for bowel complaints in children and young people and will relieve colic.

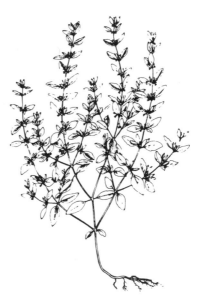

Used for centuries to promote menstruation, pennyroyal is also applied in cases of nervousness, hysteria, and the intestinal pains of colic. Toxic effects, and in one case death, have resulted from misapplication of pennyroyal in an oil form.

Pennyroyal *(Mentha pulegium)*

An herb that is solvent in alcohol or partially in water, its influences on the body include diaphoretic, diuretic, corrective, and nervine. A warm infusion of pennyroyal, used freely, will promote perspiration. It has long been used to promote menstruation. Hot footbaths taken several days before due date and two cups of pennyroyal tea, especially taken before retiring for the night, will correct scanty or suppressed flow. The herb is also used for the treatment of nervousness, hysteria, cramps, intestinal pains of colic and gripping, and as a sweating/cooling drink when treating fevers.

The infusion may be taken freely several times daily. The tincture of pennyroyal is often employed in treatment of whooping cough and spasms, taken in doses of 2 to 10 drops. The regular dosage is 1 teaspoon of the herb to 1 cup of boiling water; of the tincture, ½ to 1 fluid dram. Commonly called squaw mint, thickweed, stinking balm, and American pennyroyal, this herb grows freely throughout the country. It may be given along with other medication, and will cause such medication to have a pleasant operation.

A word of caution: In oil form, pennyroyal was responsible for the recent death of a young woman using it to cause abortion.

Pepo

Pumpkin seed or the seed of *Cucurbila pepo.* Its properties as a vermifuge are due to a resin contained in the inner covering of the embryo. Dosage of the resin is 15 grains; of the seeds, 1 ounce made into a suitable emulsion. (See *Anthelmintics.*)

Pepper, Black

The unripe fruit of *Piper nigrum,* shriveled and dried. The plant is a native of the East Indies and contains oleoresin, an alkaloid, and a volatile oil. It is a stimulant to the stomach and an irritant to the skin, and is used mainly to correct flatulence and locally for hemorrhoids. The dosage is 5 to 20 grains.

Peppermint *(Mentha x piperita)*

Very hot in nature, peppermint may be used to advantage to promote perspiration and overpower the cold. It is, however, volatile and will not retain the heat in the stomach long. In colds and slight attacks of disease, freely drinking a peppermint tea and taking bed rest aids greatly. The essence in warm water is good for treating children and will also relieve pain in the stomach and bowels. A few drops of the oil, given in warm water or on a cube of sugar, will achieve the same results.

Pepsin

The digestive ferment of gastric juice with the power of digesting proteins.

Pepsin, though present in gastric juice, is not present as such in the chief cells of the glands of the stomach, but is derived from a zymogen, propepsin or pepsinogen, when the latter is treated with hydrochloric acid. Pepsin is the chief proteolytic agent of the gastric juice and exerts its influence most energetically in the presence of hydrocholoric acid and at a temperature of about 40°C. It is employed in the treatment of dyspepsia, apepsia of infants, gastralgia, anemia, chlorosis, gastric ulcer and cancer, infantile diarrhea, vomiting during pregnancy, and in nutritive enemas. It should be administered within two or three hours after taking food. There are two preparations: saccharated pepsin and liquid pepsin.

Peptonized Food

This is indicated when the natural digestive powers are enfeebled or suspended. It may be prepared by the gastric method, using pepsin and hydrochloric acid, or by the intestinal method, making use of the extract of the pancreas with sodium bicarbonate. Probably the best solvent for an extract of pancreas is dilute spirit.

Petrissage

A method of kneading, pressing, rolling, and squeezing the tissues; principally a treatment of the muscles. Petrissage is performed with one hand, two hands, with two thumbs, or with the thumb and forefingers. In using one hand, grasp as much of the muscle as possible, squeeze, and lift while rolling and lifting and pulling it away from the bone. The process is done repeatedly, moving backward and forward or in the same direction. The thumb and finger are used in the small areas. Muscle rolling is an excellent means of manipulation. The limb is grasped with the palms of both hands and the muscles are rolled along the bone, at the same time slowly moving the hands along the limb. (See also *Massage.*)

Pharmacology

A modern term, implying the sum of scientific knowledge of drugs, which is taken to include the art of their preparation—*pharmacy*—and all that is known of their action—*pharmacodynamics.* The subject is so broad and comprehensive as to justify subdivisions.

Pharmacy
The art of preparing drugs in suitable forms for dispensing, administering, or

applying, it includes an acquaintance with much of materia medica, as well as practical and theoretical chemistry.

Pharmacognosy
The study of physical and chemical characters of drugs—the knowledge of selecting, recognizing, and identifying true and false specimens by such characteristics.

Pharmacodynamics
The study of the physiological action, power, and strength of remedial agents on living organisms.

Pharynx

The pharynx forms that part of the alimentary canal that lies behind the mouth. The seven openings into the pharynx include the two Eustachian tubes, the mouth, the larynx, and the esophagus.

Phosphates

Products of chemical activity in the cells. A healthy person eliminates from 30 to 45 grains daily. The presence of phosphates is increased by rheumatism, inflammatory disorders, nervous strain, excessively nitrogenous diet, and extensive bone disease. The amount of phosphates is decreased by kidney lesions, dyspepsia, pneumonia, exhaustion, melancholia, and during pregnancy.

Phosphorus

This salt is intimately concerned with the life and structure of the body cells. Deficiency accompanies deterioration of the bones, thus producing an accident-prone liability to fractures. Lack of this mineral also produces a loss of virility, loss of stamina, twitching muscles, and inefficient correlation of brain and muscles. Research has shown that the human brain has approximately 100 milligrams phosphorus per ounce of brain; however, this does not mean that one will become "brainier" by consuming large amounts. There is a limit to the amount of phosphorus a human can absorb. There must be at all times a ratio of 1 part calcium to every 1½ parts phosphorus, and in order to keep this ratio, a regular supply of vitamin D and, most especially, pure honey is needed. As meat has a high calcium content, those who are heavy meat eaters need more phosphorus.

Foods rich in natural phosphorus include barley, brown rice, cabbage, cheese, eggs, some fruits, halibut, kidneys, lentils, liver, milk and milk products, nuts (especially almonds, hazel nuts, peanuts, and walnuts), oats (particularly coarse-grained natural oats), okra pods, oysters, peas, peanut butter, radishes, salmon, sardines, sesame, shrimp, watercress, and wheat germ. Excellent herbal sources of phosphorus include calamus, caraway seeds, chickweed, garlic, licorice root, marigold, meadoweast flowers, and sorrel.

Phototherapy

The method of treating diseases by artificial light, which can be applied more easily than the sun's rays, with less risk and more regularity. Phototherapy rays are always available, always constant, and can be administered in quantities that give best results. Using artificial light, radiant heat can be applied for practically every disorder with excellent results.

There are many therapeutic lights or heat lamps on the market, in varying sizes from small hand lamps to the larger stand lamps. Many of the lamps are equipped with carbon-filament bulbs from 100 to 200 watts. There are also numerous types of these small lights that use ordinary incandescent bulbs placed in a socket surrounded by a reflector. (See also *Radiant Heat, Mercury Quartz Lights.*)

Phrenology

A system by which practitioners insist that they can diagnose a person's physical and mental well-being by feeling the bumps on the head.

Some credence is offered by the explanation that as a gymnast develops certain muscles that can be felt, likewise, the head develops similar telltale elevations.

Due largely to the lack of the acceptance of this practice by organized medicine, the system and research in this field has been much neglected. It generally takes two to three years to acquire expertise in this field. Modern practitioners refer to themselves as phrenologists.

Physiotherapy

A modern descriptive word for massage. The operator compels the body to act as it should normally under its own efforts. Conditions of ill or injured persons often result in bodily functions not being carried on by the body of its own volition. The object of physiotherapy is to get the body's fuel to affected areas to speed and insure healing. The massage is often accompanied by light exercise to accomplish the desired results.

Pills

Globular or ovoid masses of medicinal material, 1 to 7.5 grains, held together by an adhesive substance. These may be plain or coated with gelatin, sucrose, cocoa, tulu or silver foil (to preserve and mask odor and taste). *Enteric* pills allow passage through the stomach intact, thereby not becoming dissolved until the duodenum or intestinal tract is reached. *Concentric* pills are made of concentric layers of different ingredients to become dissolved and active at various points of the intestinal tract.

Pilocarpus *(Pilocarpus jaborandi)*

The leaflets contain acid, alkaloids, acd a volatile oil which consists primarily of pilocarpine. The dosage is 10 to 45 grains. The jaborine that is also extracted is similar to atropine in action and antagonistic to pilocarpine, but it is present only in small amounts. Pilocarpine increases secretion particularly of the skin, stimulates voluntary muscles, contracts the pupils, and sometimes causes vomiting. It is used to treat asthenic conditions such as coryza and bronchitis.

Pimenta *(Pimenta dioica)*

The immature fruit of *P. dioica* contains an aromatic, pungent, volatile oil that is used as a flavor and condiment known as allspice. It is useful in controlling flatulence and in preventing the griping of purgatives. The dosage is 10 to 40 grains.

Pine-Needle Bath

This bath can be used with good results in treating nervousness, neuritis, rheumatism, and renal and heart conditions. It stimulates the activity of the skin, and the vapor arising from the bath has a soothing effect on the linings of the air passages in the lungs. Some practitioners use pine-needle baths in place of the Nauheim Bath. The pine-needle extract can be purchased and should be added to the water according to directions. The temperature will depend on the condition being treated.

Pine-Needle Tea

In the late 1880s, an Alaskan physician, Gidebothem, was attempting to treat a case of scurvy. Having none of the standard antiscorbutics such as fresh fruit and vegetables available, he gathered some pine needles, which he made into a decoction of equal parts of needles and water. With this treatment, the patient recovered. Later investigations showed that the pine needles contained nearly as much vitamin C as orange juice. While there is little likelihood that pine needles will ever replace orange juice in the general diet, the knowledge may be useful in an emergency.

Pitch *(Pix)*

The resinous exudation of certain coniferous trees. The varieties in common use are burgundy pitch, from the Norway spruce, and *abies excelsa* and Canada pitch, from *Abies canadensis.* It is used as a base for plasters and other liquid preparations. Pitch is used to treat various chronic inflammatory conditions of the respiratory mucous membranes and, locally, chronic eczema and psoriasis.

Pituitary Body or Gland

The pituitary body, or gland, is a small, oval body attached to the base of the brain by a thin stalk. It has two lobes, the anterior, which is larger, and the posterior, which is composed chiefly of tissue and blood vessels.

The functions of the pituitary body are felt to relate mainly to the activities of the anterior lobe. The anterior lobe, through its secretion, stimulates the growth of the skeleton and associated tissues, as apparently shown by the fact that an excess of secretion in early life leads to gigantism, while a deficiency of secretion leads to defective growth and the establishment of infantilism.

The posterior lobe, through its internal secretion, assists in the regulation of carbohydrate metabolism, as shown by the fact that an excess of secretion lowers the assimilation capacity and thus leads to the development of glycosuria, while a deficiency of the secretion raises the assimilation capacity and leads to the production of fat.

The complete removal of the pituitary gland gives rise to symptoms which occur in a definite order, beginning with lowered temperature and loss of appetite, then twitching, tremors, and nervous pneumonia, and finally dyspnea and death.

Plantain *(Plantago major)*

The whole plant is considered medicinal and is solvent in water. Its influence on the body includes its action as an alterative, astringent, a diuretic, and an antiseptic. It was used by the Indians both internally and externally, and its use has been widely adopted for cooling, soothing, and healing. Plantain is acceptable to most people and is excellent for healing fresh or chronic wounds or sores. It is a superior remedy for neuralgia in dosage of 2 to 5 drops every twenty minutes. The green seed and stem, boiled in milk, will generally check diarrhea and other digestive complaints of children. The seeds have also been used for the treatment of dropsy, epilepsy, and yellow jaundice.

The clarified juice and/or seeds made into a tea or jellylike water, taken by itself or mixed with other herbs, relieves intestinal ulcers, spitting of blood, excessive menstrual flow, inflammation of the intestines and kidney, and bladder trouble, including bed-wetting and pain in the lumbar region. Plantain is also used to clear the ear of mucous, and to treat scrofula, hemorrhoids, and leucorrhea by making a strong tea and letting it steep for 30 minutes. For hemorrhoids, a tablespoon or more several times daily may be injected after bowel evacuation.

Used externally, the juice of the leaves will counteract the bite of a rattlesnake or poisonous insects if a tablespoon is taken every hour while at the same time applying bruised leaves to the wounds. It also is known to check external bleeding, erysipelas, ulcers, eczema, burns, and scalds. It can be applied to rheumaticlike pain or added in large amounts to the bath for overnight relief. Plantain is believed to be rich in vitamins C, K, and the factor T, which helps stop bleeding. It is also sometimes used to treat diabetes, dysentery, earache, inflammation of the ear, emissions, enuresis, erythema, impotence, neuralgia, polyuria, pains of the spleen, tobacco habit, toothache, delayed urination, and worms.

Plaster, Adhesive

Made of 80 parts of lead plaster, 14 parts of resin, and 6 parts of yellow wax, it is spread on muslin prepared for that purpose. Working best when heated, the plaster may be worn for weeks at a time without producing irritation. Thus it is preferable to other plasters, such as those of rubber. It offers a reliable method of dealing with leg ulcers or varicose veins, and is also used for the treatment of fractured ribs and contusions of the chest. Sprains are also often strapped with adhesive plaster. Herbs used to add healing properties to the plaster include belladonna, capsicum, menthol, and mustard.

Plaster of Paris

Gypsum cement, or calcium sulphate, mixed with water, is used for making still or immovable bandages and dressings and for the preparation of casts. An ordinary crinoline or loose-web bandage is well rubbed with a fine plaster of Paris. A thin layer of absorbent cotton or a flannel bandage is applied to the injured part and covered by the plaster bandage, which is applied wet. Additional plaster is rubbed in and the cast is thus formed and allowed to set or dry.

Poplar Bark

Both the poplars, called the white and stinking, common to the United States, are of medicinal value. The inner bark, given in tea, is used to regulate the bile and restore the digestive powers in spite of the bitter taste. A tea made from the bark is also used for treatment of headache, faintness of the stomach, and many other complaints caused by poor digestion. It is also good for obstructions of the bladder and weakness of the loins.

Potassium

A soft, silver-white metal that is a chemical element, its salts are used in fertilizers and glass, for example. Potassium is known to be one of the trace minerals necessary for the human body to perform its natural functions. Often those who are being treated with diuretics need to have potassium returned to their bodies. This sometimes can be achieved by eating oranges and bananas but is more easily regulated by using potassium in the liquid form available at most pharmacies.

Poultice (Cataplasm)

Generally employed as a means of applying heat and moisture to a certain portion of the body, poultices are sometimes medicated with anodynes, counterirritants, or disinfectants. In preparing a poultice, a thin material is made into a bag that is filled with linseed meal or other agents, and then the open end is sewn up. The bag is submerged in boiling water for a few minutes, causing the meal to swell and fill the bag. The bag should be squeezed to remove excess water, laid on the affected area, and covered with oiled silk and a bandage.

Powders

Finely pulverized drug or drugs, with or without a dilutent, such as lactose.

Priessnitz Water Cures

Vincenz Priessnitz (1799–1851), an Austrian farmer, founded the practice of hydrotherapy. After much research, he arrived at the conclusion that bacteria dislike cold much more than heat, since cold renders unsuitable breeding conditions. One of the Priessnitz treatments, which is followed fairly widely in Europe, is called winding. A wet towel is wound around the nude patient. Around this a layer of nettles is laid, followed by a thick blanket which keeps the water against the patient. Treatments such as these are given to patients in bed. Honey-sweetened herbal teas are frequently served, and the patient's feet and hands are kept warm. The patient must have evacuated the bladder and bowels first. The windings are usually changed hourly. Temperature readings are taken every 30 minutes to make sure the patient doesn't become too cold. This treatment should be applied only by those properly trained in Priessnitz's methods. Oak bark is often used in windings for the treatment of weeping eczema, and chamomile flowers for wounds that have not healed well, inflammations, and so on. The calamus is used for circulatory troubles of arms and legs, and oat straw for rheumatic ills and chills. (See also *Kneipp Water Therapy, Sauna Bath.*)

Proteins

These are necessary in order to build blood, muscles, glands, nerves, and other tissues of the body. Some of the principal foods containing protein are meat, eggs, fish, cheese, beans, peas, lentils, and nuts. Proteins, when taken in excess of the actual needs of the body for tissue building, have a tendency to produce autointoxication. These excesses place a tremendous burden on the liver and kidneys in their work of eliminating the poisonous waste from unutilized food protein. Unless one is doing strenuous work or exercise, protein intake should be small. Those suffering disorders brought on by overindulgence should adopt a low-protein diet.

Psychic Surgery (Orificial, Bloodless, Philippine)

This surgery is performed by twenty-six recognized "surgeons" in the Philippine Islands and a few other isolated regions in the world. The practice, believed by these surgeons to come from a "higher power," involves the actual opening of the patient's body through power of the mind only, and the removal of anything that is causing trouble. This ranges from blood clots to malignant tumors. The suffering and infirm travel to the Philippines by the thousands yearly for treatment for which the surgeons make no charge, although "free-will" donations are encouraged.

Psychoanalysis

The professional practice of diagnosing and treating a patient suffering from any one of a large number of mental illnesses or psychoses. Procedures include evaluation and, depending on the seriousness or the nature of the illness, measures of treatment range from counseling to drug therapy and institutionalization.

Psychometry

Although many people scoff, some spiritualists are possessed of remarkable talents which have become known as psychometry. Some are handed an object belonging to someone totally unknown to them, who is often not even in the room. The psychometrist (often a woman) closes her eyes, holds the object carefully, and describes with remarkable accuracy the physical characteristics of the person—sex, age, color of hair, eyes, shape of features, and so forth. Psychometrists are also capable of giving full diagnoses of physical diseases and difficulties as well as emotional and spiritual problems that face the unknown person. They are rarely wrong, and are often used with amazing results by police departments to find missing persons, wanted criminals, and so on. Theirs is a natural, radiesthetic sense on a very high spiritual plane (see also *Radiesthesia*). Most gifted persons work entirely without payment because they feel that if they made a living from it, the psychic gift would disappear and never return. Perhaps the best known psychometrist of recent times was Edgar Cayce.

Psychosomatic Healing

The relationship of mind and body is a very close one. When they are faced with adversity, humans react with the "flight or fight" syndrome, physically or mentally. Complicated human emotions such as self-respect, frustration, conflict, unhappiness, and feelings of inadequacy may cause psychosomatic illness. Disappointments, hurts, frustrations, and violent emotions are often turned inward—toward the body and its delicate functions. Anger and frustration can, if they are strong enough, change the chemical constitution of the stomach acids in a matter of minutes. The blood and lymphatic secretions of the body are affected by the mind, and from their behavior, the muscles and even the bones take their health or ill health.

Research has shown how emotional behavior can lead to constant tensing of the muscles and thus to fibrositis, rheumatism, and arthritic complaints. Insecurity or the feeling of having let oneself down can induce angina pectoris, migraine, asthma, and coronary thrombosis. Those who cannot cope adequately with social problems are likely to get ill. Those who are frequently ill should study this approach to healing; treatment methods vary, but often include counseling, diet improvement, physical exercise, massage, manipulation, and similar modalities.

Pulse

Pulse refers to the rate, rhythm, and condition of arterial walls. The normal rate of the pulse is 76 beats per minute for a male and 80 for a female. At birth, it is from 120 to 130. To take the pulse, the patient should be seated. Place the four fingers on the left radial artery of the patient, with the index finger nearest the patient's hand. The pulse should always be taken at the wrist, since by doing so, aneurysms may often be detected. Increased pulse rate may result from excitement, exercise, use of certain drugs such as aconite and digitalis, fever, shock, exophthalmic goiter, pressure on the base of the brain, and organic or heart disease. A slow pulse is seen in jaundice, atheroma, lesions of the cerebral centers and fatty degeneration.

Alterations of rhythm are seen in an intermittent or an irregular pulse. This may be the result of tobacco use, overeating, constipation, or disease of the stomach, liver, or kidneys. Irregular pulse is often found in organic heart disease. The alterations in volume, strength, and tension may be felt by the fingers when taking the rate or by the means of a *sphygmograph*. A *dicrotic* pulse occurs when the first impulse is quickly followed by another impulse or secondary wave. The *waterhammer* pulse is characterized by a short, sharp, strong pulse which seems to collapse under the finger.

Purgatives (See *Cathartics*)

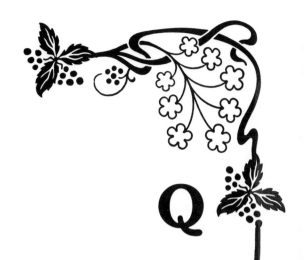

Quassia *(Picrasma excelsa)*

Raspings or chips of a yellowish-white color from the wood of the *Picrasma excelsa,* a large tree of Jamaica and other West Indian islands.

Quassia is inodorous but has an intensely bitter taste. It is used as a bitter tonic in atonic dyspepsia and as an enema (3½ teaspoons of decoction to a pint of water) against seatworms or threadworms. A bitter tonic is as follows: extract of nux vomica, 4 grams; extract of quassia, 20 grams. Make into 20 pills and give one pill three times daily following meals. The infusion is drunk to stimulate aversion to alcoholic beverages.

Quinine

A finely crystalline or amorphous white alkaloid obtained from various species of Cinchona. It is odorless, very bitter, and alkaline in reaction (see *Alkalies*). It is a valuable tonic, antiseptic, antipyretic, and antiperiodic. It is particularly valuable in the treatment of malaria, in which condition it is both prophylactic and curative. It also is used as an antipyretic in septic fevers and typhus, acute rheumatism, acute tonsillitis, neuralgia, and certain skin diseases. Large doses of quinine often produce a sense of fullness and constriction in the head, cerebral anemia, pallor, tinnitus, vertigo, staggering gait, deafness, and dilated pupils. The principal preparations are obtained by prescription while under a physician's care.

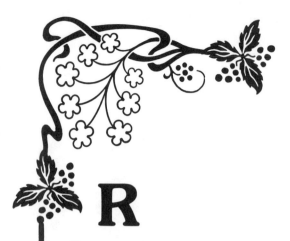

R

Radiant Heat

A very penetrating type of heat. It helps break up congestion, stimulates the circulation, and is soothing to the nerves. Aches and pains from rheumatism, neuritis, neuralgia, and so on can be relieved by a few minutes' use of these therapeutic lamps.

Radiesthesia

A method of diagnosing and treating illnesses through the use of devices that respond to vibration. A response to such vibrations is inborn in the individual; the tools employed have no value in themselves. Radiesthesia includes dowsing, pendulum, and similar modes, although most practitioners use a pendulum. Because magnetism is a factor, the radiesthesist must remove all metal jewelry and turn off all electrical appliances. The practitioner must also be trained not to intervene in the process with his or her own thought patterns. The scope of what may be accomplished is seemingly unlimited. Although there are some forty distinguished pendulum movements, basically there are the positive, negative,and neutral positions, or reactions. It was discovered in Europe at the turn of the twentieth century that there are distinctly different results for healthy and sick organisms and people. Radiesthesia is an excellent method by which to determine which of the various healing arts is most suitable for an individual. Radiesthesia speeds up all forms of diagnosis, and, since the exact number of vibrations differs in each condition, an expert has less chance of making a mistake.

An electronic version of radiesthesia, called radionics, was also developed. Some doctors have acquired modern, computer-type machines for their own use. One of the drawbacks of all radiesthetic and radionic work is that if a practitioner becomes in any way subjectively involved in the matter being examined, efficiency is lost. In the hands of an expert, radionics is remarkably accurate; without proper training or natural ability, it is almost useless.

Red Clover *(Trifolium pratense)*

Common in pastures, lawns, and roadsides throughout the United States and Canada, the medicinal parts are the blossoms and leaves, which are solvent in boiling water or alcohol. The efficacy of red clover to counteract a scrofulous disposition and as antidote for cancer results from its high content of lime, silica, and other earthy salts.

Possessing very soothing and pleasant-tasting properties, red clover is used in the treatment of malignant ulcers, scrofula, indolent sores, burns, whooping cough, and various spasms, and bronchial and renal conditions. The warm tea is very soothing to the nerves. A fine formula for the above is equal parts of blue violet, burdock, yellow dock, dandelion, rock rose and golden seal. Obviously red clover may be used alone or in combination. The dosage, taken as an infusion, is 1 teaspoon of red clover to 1 cup of boiling water, steeped for 30 minutes or more. Take 4 to 6 cups a day. Children's doses are somewhat less. The dosage taken as a tincture is 5 to 30 drops in water, according to age and purpose. Taken externally, red clover has been used successfully as a salve for the removal of external cancers and ulcers. A tea, made fresh daily, is also helpful to bathe the affected part.

Red Raspberry *(Rubus idaeus)*

An excellent herb, used medicinally for canker, and the leaves, when made into a strong tea, will relax and treat bowel complaints of children. It is one of the best things available for women in labor, when a strong tea with a little sweetener will provide a natural regulator. If the pains are untimely, it will subdue them. When the child is born, some of the tea with sugar and milk in it prevents sore mouth. And the tea is good to wash sore nipples with, and also to increase milk flow. A poultice made with the tea and cracker or slippery elm bark is very good for burns or scalds; if the skin is off, applying red raspberry as a poultice or washing with the tea will harden the area and stop smarting. Solvent in water or alcohol, red raspberry has been a long-established remedy for dysentery and diarrhea, especially in infants. It is a mild, pleasant, soothing way to remove cankers from mucous membranes, at the same time toning the tissue involved. It is also much used for relief of urethral irritation and is soothing to the kidneys, urinary tract, and ducts.

Reflexology (Zone therapy)

An ancient form of Chinese therapy that has recently been rediscovered in the United States. For thousands of years, it has been felt that the hands are maps of an individual's character. Likewise, it is ancient knowledge that the feet are maps of an individual's state of physical balance. Everyone knows that the soles of the feet are very sensitive. Through them, the body is connected with the earth. Although wearing shoes insulates us from the therapeutic value of being "earthed," or connected to earth energy, both positively and negatively, the fact that we do wear shoes makes our feet more sensitive and amenable to foot, or zone, therapy.

There is a correspondence in this sense between the principle of acupuncture and the principle of reflexology. For specific areas of the soles of the feet (see chart) seem to relate to individual organic functions. If an organ loses its state of balance with the whole organism, a sensitive nodule can form in its specific area. Practiced manipulation or massage of this spot will lead to quick relief of the imbalance, just as needles inserted or manipulated in the specific acupuncture point corresponding to the organ will bring the organ into balance.

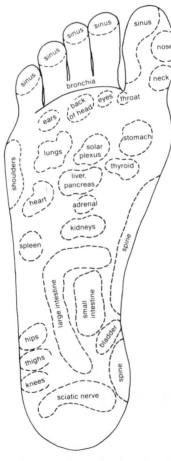

The foot is divided into "zones," which correspond to various organs and parts of the body. A slight pressure massage is applied with the tips of the thumbs and fingers; this breaks up deposits of calcium and restores free flow of energy to the corresponding organ.

This form of manipulation of the feet can be done by anyone, although there are persons who specialize in foot reflexology. The diagnostic use of reflexology by physicians includes noting any areas where firm pressing causes extreme pain. The corresponding area of the body is then investigated for possible chronic disease.

Specialists claim many conditions are helped by reflexology of both feet and hands, such as stomach troubles, sexual problems, and appendicitis; but they do not claim responsibility for curing a disease, as this is up to the body itself, which is stimulated by the treatment to engage its self-healing mechanisms.

Reichian Therapeutics

Throughout Europe and in some large American cities, the Reichian form of healing is gaining adherents. The basic theory is that all mental stresses, anxieties, neuroses, and emotional conflicts are expressed unconsciously in the body. Loneliness, anger, secretiveness, suspicion, and inability to trust or love others all can manifest themselves as various illnesses, say the therapists, and they work upon the body to produce reactions in the physical medium which relate to the emotional state. As an emotional release is effected, the relationship of mind and body is corrected. The theory is closely related to the psychosomatic approach of psychology. Some practitioners apply their attention to the feet and reflex areas of the body. (See *Reflexology.*)

Resins

Powders obtained by exhausting the vegetable herb with alcohol, and precipitating the tincture by adding water; they contain all the principles soluble in alcohol and insoluble in water.

Respiration

The process by which oxygen is introduced into and carbon dioxide removed from the body. The respiratory apparatus includes: lungs and the air passages leading into them, nasal chambers, mouth, pharynx, larynx, and trachea, and the throat and its associated structures. The continuous recurrence of inspiration and expiration brings about the ventilation necessary for the normal exchange of gases between the blood and the air. Inspiration is an active process, the result of the expansion of the thorax, whereby atmospheric air is introduced into the lungs. Expiration is a partially passive process, the result of the recoil of the elastic walls of the thorax and the recoil of the elastic tissue of the lungs whereby air is to be expelled. The number of respirations per minute varies with age and condition: during the first year of life, there are 44 changes per minute; from thirty to fifty years of age, 17 per minute. During sleep, however, the volume varies with ordinary inspiration, ordinary expiration, and both forced inspiration and expiration. After the expiration of the reserve volume, there is yet remaining an unknown volume of air in the lungs, which cannot be displaced by effort but resides permanently in the alveoli and bronchial tubes, though this air is constantly being exchanged.

Rest Cure

This treatment is usually prescribed for restoration of the vitality of the feeble or overworked. It is effected by a combination of isolation from friends, rest in bed for from four to six weeks, and excessive or forced feeding, together with the thorough use of massage and various forms of electrotherapy. The cases best suited for this treatment are those in which the enfeebled condition has resulted from an infectious disease such as pneumonia, those of chronic dypepsia, malarial toxemia, neurasthenia, spinal irritation, and so forth.

Retina

The innermost or nervous tunic of the eye. It is a delicate, grayish, transparent membrane formed by a membranous expansion of the optic nerve elements. It extends from the termination of that nerve nearly as far forward as the ciliary processes.

Rheum (See *Rhubarb*)

Rhubarb *(Rheum officinale)*

The root of *Rheum officinale* or other species of *Rheum,* it is used as a cholagogue, a purgative stomachic, and an astringent. It is valuable as a laxative in children, and is particularly useful in treating diarrhea, due to the astringent afteraffects. The principle preparation is the tincture in doses of 3 to 4 drops in, with, and as a tea.

For treatment of summer diarrhea in children, make a combination of 6 teaspoons aromatic syrup of rhubarb, 2 teaspoons sodium bicarbonate, and enough peppermint water to make a half-pint. A child aged from four to six years should be given a teaspoonful every three hours.

Riedlin System

Named after Dr. Gustav Riedlin, the system treats illness by means of fasting. The theory is that the life force is not simply physical-chemical but, essentially, is also mental-spiritual. Not just a machine that produces energy by food combustion, the body is also a living force depending upon all permeating cosmic energy. This cosmic energy is equally contained in food itself, particularly in unheated fruits and vegetables.

Riedlin reasoned that if the purpose of food is to replace worn-out cells, furnish energy for mind and body, and create warmth, then logically with an increase of food there should be more warmth and energy. But his experience showed this is not the case. In fact, the opposite was noted; by eating less food and taking more rest, more strength would accumulate. For Riedlin, fasting was a natural process presented by nature, only waiting to be acknowledged by humans.

Rikli's Sunshine Cure

Arnold Rikli, who died in 1906, spent his life advocating exposing one's body to the sun to improve health.

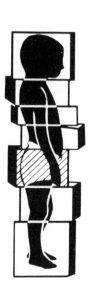
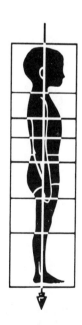

This symbolic outline of a human body represents the corrected relation of the segments of the body before and after rolfing.

Rolfing

A method of deep, soft-tissue manipulation developed by Ida Rolf in the

1950s. As a self-treatment for adhesions, the patient lies on the back with both legs drawn up. With all five fingers of the left hand, the abdominal region is deeply manipulated in the search for tight bands or other constrictive involvements. With the flat part of the right thumb, the left hand firmly presses downward and outward to a slight degree. Adhesive tissues, being inelastic, will "give" by the pressure of the right thumb, thus releasing their hold on affected tissues. The presence of pockets or diverticula is felt to be the direct result of adhesions. Usually a series of ten "Rolfing sessions" is scheduled, proceeding to each region of the body until all tissues assume elastic consistencies. Adhesions formed as the result of surgery have developed to such a great extent that they cannot be removed by this manipulative technique. However, so-called spiderweb adhesions, which result from blows, injuries, or inflammations, do respond to this treatment.

Royal Jelly

A special elaborated honey composed of honey and pollen, worked upon by the bees until it becomes ultranutritious and assimilable: the food of the queen bees.

Russian Bath

The application of hot vapor or steam at a temperature ranging from 105 to 145° F. The patient is allowed to remain in the steam-heated area from ten to twenty minutes, after which a hot shower is given and the body is then massaged. The body is then scraped, brushed, showered, and cooled gradually, dried, and allowed to rest for from one to several hours.

Salt Glow (Salt Bath)

Given to feeble persons whose skin and circulation are weak or dormant, the salt glow consists of moistened salt rubbed briskly over the entire body. After the salt glow, the entire body should be showered or sprayed off. This treatment should not be used when there is any disease or condition affecting the skin.

Samuels Therapy

A high-frequency short-wave irradiation treatment for cancer which restores the hormone balance by stimulating the endocrine glands.

The theory is that a causative factor of cancer is the dysfunctioning of the endocrine system, particularly the pituitary gland, which causes an imbalance between the thyrotropic and gonadotropic hormones, both of which are produced by the pituitary—an excess of the thyrotropic (growth accelerating) hormone is secreted, while the gonadotropic (growth-retarding) hormone is deficient.

See the book *Endogenous Endocrine Therapy—Including the Causal Treatment of Cancer,* by Jules Samuels, M.D., oncologist and endocrinologist, and director of Centrale Inrichting Voor de Samuels-Therapie, Plantage Parklaan 20, Amsterdam, Holland. His technique is fully set forth in this book, published by N. V. Cycloscoop, Amsterdam.

Sandalwood *(Santalum album)*

The wood and oil of this small tree, common to India, are used internally in bronchitis, gonorrhea, and cystitis, and are also employed as an expectorant, a perfume, and for coloring and dyeing.

Its medicinal properties are due to an astringent oil, santal, which is usually given in doses of from 5 to 15 drops, depending upon the condition to be treated.

Sanguinaria (See *Bloodroot*)

Santonica (American Wormseed) *Chenopodium ambrosioides*

This plant is indigenous to Mexico and South America, but also grows naturally as far north as Missouri and New England. Its medicinal properties are due to a crystalline principle, santonin, a very efficient anthelmintic against the roundworm.

The part used is the flowering head, which, because of its low toxicity and ease of administration, is perhaps one of the most widely used medicines for worms, especially in children. As with most vermifuges, administration is usually preceded by catharsis (see *Cathartics*) and fasting. Large doses produce a yellow color in the urine and can be toxic. The usual dosage of the fluidextract is from ½ to 1 dram.

Sarsaparilla (Similax officinalis)

There are several species of the sarsaparilla—red sarsaparilla, small spikenard, spignet, qual, and quill—which are indigenous to Central America, Mexico, northern South America and the.West Indies. The American sarsaparilla is a member of the ginseng family. The roots being the part most used commer-

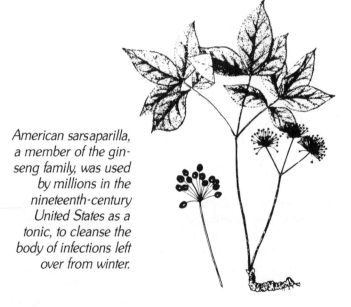

American sarsaparilla, a member of the ginseng family, was used by millions in the nineteenth-century United States as a tonic, to cleanse the body of infections left over from winter.

cially acts as an alterative, a diuretic, a demulcent, a stimulant, and an antiscorbutic. The texture of the sarsaparilla root is mucilaginous; it has scarcely any odor.

In the mid-1800s, sarsaparilla was something of a national phenomenon in the United States. It was used as a spring tonic to eliminate poisons from the blood and to purify the system from the leftover infections of the winter. It has long been used to treat rheumatism, gout, skin eruptions, ringworm, scrofula, internal inflammation, colds, catarrh, fever, and gas in the stomach and bowels. Given as an antidote in cases of poisoning, it causes vomiting, and can be drunk afterward as a relieving and cleansing tea. It has also been employed to treat infants affected with venereal disease: the pustules of the sores are washed with a tea, and the powdered form is then given in the food.

The normal dose of sarsaparilla is 1 ounce of the root boiled in 1 pint of water and taken in small amounts three times a day. For colds, it is given in syrup form, 1 teaspoon to 1 tablespoonful a day, depending on the age and condition of the patient. Externally, it is used in ointment form for swelling, rheumatic pain, boils, and carbuncles.

Sassafras *(Sassafras officinalis)*

The generic name for three species of tree, one of which is native to the United States and grows from Maine through Texas and Florida. It is well recognized by its agreeable fragrance, credited in the 1884 book *Trees and Shrubs of Massachusetts* as having aided Columbus in his discovery of the Americas.

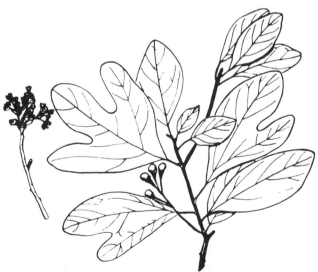

Indians taught early American settlers the many healing uses of sassafras. Its effects in thinning and purifying the blood make it a popular spring tonic. Sassafras is also used by women for painful menstrual cramps and to ease childbirth.

As the wind-swept, pleasant odor of sassafras reached the ships, he was able to persuade his nearly mutinous men that land was near. The Indians taught the early American settlers the many curative powers of the bark, roots, and oils of sassafras.

Its effect of "thinning" and purifying the blood accounts for its reputation as a spring renovator to the system. It is used as an expectorant, a corrective in rheumatism, for varicose ulcers, and to relieve painful menstruation cramps, as well as during the afterpains of childbirth and as a combative against the narcotic effects of alcohol in the system. The oil is often used to cure toothache and as an ingredient in liniment, providing a common application for bruises and swellings.

Because of its particularly agreeable taste and odor, sassafras is often used with other compounds to improve their taste. It is boiled in water, usually 1 ounce of the crushed or chip bark to 1 pint of water.

Sauna Bath

This therapeutic procedure was developed in Finland. It consists of subjecting the body to steam-saturated, overheated rooms at regular intervals.

A true Finnish sauna is made by putting chips of birch logs into an oven, igniting them, and placing large stones over the coals, over which cold water is poured. The firewood is replenished from time to time, and cold water is occasionally added to the rocks to keep up the steam in the air. A roof vent is kept open.

The sauna-bath temperature is kept between 212 and 250° F. The initial bath should not last more than five minutes for adults, and less for children under five. This can gradually be increased to twenty minutes, in increments of five minutes. It is customary to follow the stay in the bath with an icy cold shower or a plunge into a lake or stream. The sauna bath may also be accompanied by a slight stroking massage with a birch-leaf *vihta* (a bunch of twigs bound together) or a similar bunch of juniper pine needles.

Saw Palmetto *(Serenoa repens)*

The nut of the native American plant yields a volatile oil which is sedative, nutritive (due to the presence of glucose), and tonic. It is similar in effect to sandalwood, but somewhat milder in its effect upon the respiratory system. Dose of the fluidextract is ½ to 1 teaspoon.

Scales, Lamellae

Thin scales, disks, or plates of medicinal substances; in England, restricted to gelatin and glycerin, to be dropped into the eye, each weighing 1/50 grains (.0013 grams).

Scammony *(Convolvulus scammonia)*

The root of this southwestern Asiatic plant is made into a juice which is dehydrated for medicinal applications. It is a drastic cathartic and should not be used when there is inflammation of the bowels.

The primary application of this plant is in homeopathy. Another species, jalap bindweed (*Ipomea purga*), is similarly purgative and cathartic, and is used in the treatment of constipation, and colic; in combination with other herbs, such as rhubarb, it speeds their action. Another member of the bindweed family, *Convolvulus batatas,* is grown for its tuberous root, which is known by the common name "sweet potato."

Schlenz Cure

A German woman, Maria Schlenz, developed this form of hydrotherapy, which became known as the "cure for the incurables."

The method is based on artifically increasing the body temperature to the point that a mild fever is induced. To accomplish this, the patient is totally immersed, including the head (except for nose, eyes and mouth), in a tub of hot water. The temperature of the water is, at first, equal to or slightly above normal body temperature, and is gradually increased over a period of 20 to 30 minutes, with the temperature of the patient monitored until it reaches an elevation of 2 to 3 degrees above normal.

After this immersion, there is copious perspiration, and the patient is removed from the bath, wrapped in several layers of light blankets, and left to rest or sleep while the process of perspiration continues to completion, or about two hours.

Those who follow this therapy in Europe claim that a hormone is invoked during the fever that produces remarkable healing results. The bath should not be performed more than once a week.

Schott Treatment

A systematic use of saline baths of specific strength and temperature, along with a series of resisted movements. The treatment originated in Bad Nauheim,

Germany, where natural salt springs heavily charged with carbonic gas are located. For specifics of the treatment, see *Nauheim Bath.*

Schroth Therapy

Although not a medical doctor, Johann Schroth (1798–1856) learned from "nature," in his native Germany, a system of cure so effective that he was given a license to practice by the prestigious German medical profession.

After observing animals abstaining from all food during periods of illness, Schroth himself, after being injured by being kicked in the leg by a horse, engaged in a prolonged fast, which resulted in a complete and rapid recovery.

The Schroth Fasting Cure gained wide acceptance throughout Europe. It favors dry foods and strict control over the amount of fluid intake. Schroth also employed forms of damp hot packs over affected organs, and generally produced a total restoration of the circulatory and eliminative systems.

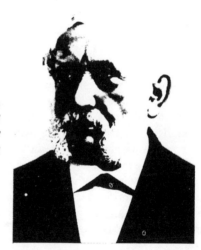

Wilhelm H. Schuessler, the German chemist, identified the twelve "tissue salts" present in every human cell in a state of health.

Schuessler Tissue Salts

Wilhelm Heinrich Schuessler, a German physiological chemist and physicist, synthesized the work of several contemporary scientists in the early nineteenth century and identified twelve "tissue salts," which he found were present in every healthy human cell.

In order to be absorbed by the body, therapeutic doses of these salts were made in minute concentrations in the same way that homeopathic remedies are made.

The twelve salts identified by Schuessler are: calcium fluoride; calcium phosphate; calcium sulphate; ferrous phosphate; potassium chloride; potassium phosphate; potassium sulphate; sodium chloride; sodium phosphate; sodium sulphate; magnesium phosphate, and silic oxide.

This method requires a practitioner trained both in identifying deficiencies of these salts and arriving at proper dosages. Generally speaking, one or more of the salts in prepared form (usually on a fructose base) are taken in doses of 4 to 10 tablets at intervals of thirty minutes. Homeopaths make considerable use of the biochemic, or Schuessler tissue salts, in their treatment, either alone or in combination with other remedies and procedures.

Semen

A fluid generated in the male, made up of secretions from the testicles, vesiculae seminates, and prostatic and urethral glands. At each orgasm, approximately one to five cubic centimeters of the whitish, mucilaginous fluid having a characteristic odor are ejaculated. Semen contains the reproductive element called sperm.

Senega *(Polygala senega)*

Also called Seneca snakeroot, it is a root which acts as a diuretic and an expectorant. It is used in bronchitis, asthenic pneumonia, and asthma. In large doses, it acts as a gastrointestinal irritant. The principal preparations are the fluidextract (dose, 10–30 drops), the syrup, and the compound syrup.

Senna (*Cassia angustifolia*)

The leaves, which are soluble in water and alcohol, are used as a laxative, an anthelmintic, vermifuge, and a cathartic. Senna sometimes causes griping effects, which can be modified by combining senna leaves with one of the aromatic herbs such as ginger, anise, caraway, fennel, or coriander. It may also be used in combination with spigelia.

It should not be used in cases of inflammation of the stomach. It is also of use in the treatment of colic in infants, exhaustion, nitrogenous waste, sleeplessness, and sneezing, in combination with heat. For treating constipation, the buds are often preferred, mixed with oils. This may be used repeatedly without side effects.

Skin diseases and pimples are treated with a paste made of the dried leaves mixed with vinegar. Senna is further used in the treatment of biliousness, gout, and rheumatism, in the form of decoctions, infusions, powders, and confections. It should not be administered for fever, piles, menorrhagia, prolapse of the rectum or uterus, or in pregnancy. The dosage is 1 to 2 tablespoonsful of the tincture; 10 to 20 grains of powder; and ½ to 1 cup of the infusion steeped for 30 minutes.

Shower Baths

As opposed to immersion in water, a bath consisting of water sprayed in numerous jets from above the patient's head in varying temperatures. The impact of the water on the skin affects the nervous system. Cold shower baths are recommended only for those who do not suffer from high blood pressure or weakened heart conditions, as the colder water shocks the nerves and raises the blood pressure.

Patients in less vigorous health can begin by taking baths with water that is reduced in force and more tepid in temperature. Generally, the coldest shower bath should last only about 2 to 3 minutes.

Sialogogues

Saliva-producing drugs that are divided into two groups, depending on their action in the body. Topical sialogogues work by reflex stimulation and are chiefly acids and alkalies, chloroform, mustard, ginger, tobacco, cubebs, capsicum, horseradish, and rhubarb. General sialogogues act through a systemic influence on the glands or their secretory nerves. They are pilocarpus (jaborandi), muscarine, physostigma, mercurials, iodine compounds, antimonials, tobacco, ipececuanha, and stillingia.

Silicon

Essential in the body for maintaining the alkaline balance of tissues, silicon facilitates quick nerve reactions, gives hardness to bones and teeth, and aids in healthy eyesight. The eyes contain a great deal more silicon naturally than do the muscles of the human body, and older persons are generally found to have about 20 percent less silicon in the body than younger persons.

Deficiency of silicon apparently results in speedy exhaustion, nervous debility, and tendency to suffer from cold feet and hands, and is thought to effect the loss of hair.

Silicon is usually found in horsetail grass, comfrey, dandelions, herb nettle, and hound's tongue. Foods containing silicon are artichokes, asparagus, barley, cabbage, celery, cucumbers, leeks, lettuce, liver, milk, mushrooms, nuts, oats, spinach, strawberries, sunflower seeds, tomatoes, and turnips.

Silver

A metal of brilliant white luster, malleable, ductile, and generally administered as salts in cases of dyspepsia, chronic gastritis, gastric ulcer, chronic dysentery, diarrhea from asthma and typhoid fever, chronic spinal inflammations, and epilepsy.

The nitrate of silver is used as a caustic, an excitant, an astringent and a hemostatic.

Continued overuse of silver salts may result in gastrointestinal catarrh, uremia, albuminuria, fatty degeneration of the viscera, and impairment of the nervous system, and often results in the appearance of a salt-colored line along the margin of the gums, along with discoloration of the skin and mucous membranes. Common table salt is the chemical antidote for silver poisoning.

Sinusoidal Current

Sinusoidal current is a smoothly alternating current of low voltage and high amperage. Properly administered, the waves are slow, rapid, or surging, depending upon the application. Sinusoidal currents are considered to be similar in effect, but much superior in application, to faradic current. Sinusoidal current is employed especially to evoke muscular contraction so that toxic matters may be expelled, flow of lymph increased, and muscular adhesions loosened.

Sinusoidal current is the main form of applying *electric baths.* The bathtub is filled with warm water—about 95° F. The patient lies in the tub; one electrode is placed at the head of the tub and the other at the foot. Electrodes must be insulated from the tub and must not touch the patient. The bath usually lasts about fifteen minutes and is done under a doctor's care only. (See also *Electrotherapy.*)

Sitz Bath

Baths, of either hot or cold water, designed for sitting rather than reclining of the patient. The level of water should be high enough to cover the hips and pelvic region. The bath container is such that one is immersed from the navel to the knees only. Hot sitz baths are used to relieve pain and inflammation of the reproductive organs and other organs of the pelvic region. Generally lasting from ten to fifteen minutes in water as hot as can be comfortably borne, they increase the circulation through the covered area.

The cold-water sitz bath is used for its invigorating effect on the spine and pelvic organs. The patient should remain in water from 50 to 65 degrees in temperature for about three to ten minutes. Often the feet of the patient are placed in a small tub of hot or warm water during the cold bath. This bath may be taken two to three times weekly, or more often by persons in good health.

Patients of lowered vitality can best use the alternate hot and cold baths, employing two separate tubs and beginning by immersion in the hot water for 3 to 4 minutes and then changing to the cold tub for 1 to 2 minutes only. This should be continued three or four times and should always end with the cold-water bath.

Skin

Made up of the epidermis or cuticle (the first five layers from the body surface) and the derma or cutis vera (composed of a papillary layer above and a reticular layer below), often called the true skin.

The epidermis contains neither vessels nor nerves, and its cells are disorganized in a laminated arrangement—those on the top are flat and dry, growing rounder and softer in the central portion, and becoming almost columnar and softest in the deepest layer.

The derma is a highly organized, tough, yet elastic tissue serving to protect the body parts underneath, to perform the functions of excretion and absorption, and to act as the chief seat of the sense of touch. The derma consists of connective tissue, elastic fibers, blood vessels, lymphatics, and nerves.

Skullcap *(Scutellaria lateriflora)*

The whole herb is medicinal and soluble in alcohol or boiling water. It is employed with success as a nervine and an antispasmodic, and is slightly as-

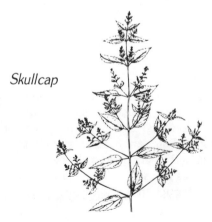

Skullcap

tringent. Because of its action in the cerebrospinal centers, it is a valuable remedy for controlling nervous irritation. It has been known to render the patient free of disturbance in many cases of hydrophobia. This is also true in cases of insomnia, excitability, and restlessness.

Skunk Cabbage *(Symplocarpus foetidus)*

The root of this vegetable, which looks like a cabbage and has a disagreeable odor, is used as a remedy. When it is dried and ground into a powder, it may be taken in a sweetened tea or made into a syrup. It may also be taken by the teaspoonful with honey morning or night. It is useful in the treatment of asthma, cough, breathing difficulty, and all disorders of the lungs. It is a stimulant, an expectorant, antispasmodic, a diuretic, and has a slight narcotic influence.

Slippery Elm Bark *(Ulmus fulva)*

The inner bark of the elm may be used to advantage in many ways. There are several species of elm common to this country. The one with the brittle bark is the best for medicinal purposes. The bark should be peeled, the outside dross shaved off, dried, and ground into a powder. If used internally, add a teaspoonful in a teacup to a teaspoonful of sugar, and mix and add a little cold water. Mix well and add hot water until a jelly thick enough to eat with a spoon forms. A teaspoonful taken at a time is excellent to heal soreness in the throat, stomach, and bowels caused by canker. More water may be added and the medicinal properties taken in tea form.

Small Intestine

Connecting the pyloric opening of the stomach and the colon, or large intestine, is about 20 feet of coiled tissue containing intestinal, pancreatic, and biliary juices having enzymes that act to break down food taken into the body. The small intestine is divided into the duodenum, the jejunum, and the ileum; it processes all the nutrients in the stomach. The numerous membranes of the small intestine contain villi which facilitate the passing of undigested material or fecal matter into the colon for excretion.

Intestinal juices contain the enzyme erepsin, which reduces proteins and peptones into aminos acids; and invertase and maltase, which change the various sugars into simple sugars.

The bile salts assist in the emulsification of fats and exert an antiseptic effect on the whole intestine. About 1 pound of bile juice, 1½ pounds of pancreatic juice, and 2½ pounds of bile are secreted every twenty-four hours.

Snake Root (See *Senega*)

Sodium

A natural component of the body, found in all the fluids of the body, especially the gastric juices. Its primary function is that of helping rid the body of acids; it is also an agent in the speedy coagulation of the blood.

Sodium deficiency is known to cause cramping and slow healing of scratches and wounds. The body's natural sodium is lost in great quantities through perspiration during strenuous activity, while the minimal loss through urination is well controlled by the kidneys.

Many persons, in an effort to restore sodium to the body, consume extra quantities of common table salt, or sodium chloride, which is not to be confused with natural sodium. One gram of sodium chloride can cause the body to retain 70 grams of fluid, or 1 teaspoonful can keep about a quart of unnecessary liquid in the body. Sea salt contains more of the necessary balance of magnesium and potassium than table salt, and there are also balanced salts on the market which are nontoxic, since the minerals they contain have been matched to the quantities that occur naturally in the human body.

Foods containing natural sodium are carrots, celery, cheddar cheese, raw herring, lentils, nuts, oats, spinach, and raw steak. Herbs rich in natural sodium are beets, black willow, carrageen moss, chives, cleavers, devil's bit, fennel seed, meadowsweet, mistletoe, nettles, rest harrow, shepherd's purse, sorrel, watercress, and waywort.

Spearmint *(Mentha spicata)*

Often referred to as the garden mint, it is chiefly used for culinary purposes. Its properties resemble those of peppermint, being stimulant, carminative, and antispasmodic, although it is less powerful in effect. Its taste, which is pleasanter than that of peppermint, adds much to the flavor of many foods and aids in the digestion as well.

Spearmint is most often given medicinally in the form of oil on sugar or with a small amount of water, and is also drunk as a pleasant beverage to aid cases of fevers and inflammatory diseases. The infusion is made by pouring a pint of boiling water on 1 ounce of the dried herb. The strained liquid is then consumed in small glassfuls and is used to relieve hiccup, flatulence, nausea, and vomiting.

Much cooking is done with spearmint in its dried or fresh chopped form, and various foods are enhanced by spearmint in the form of jelly, sauce, and vinegar.

Spigelia *(Spigelia marilandica)*

Also called pink root, S. *marilandica* is the root of a plant once collected by American Indians for sale to white traders. The Indians used it largely for worms, it being an active vermifuge.

In great use today, it is often administered to children in the fluidextract, in powder, and combined with senna, fennel or wheatgrass. It has a potentially narcotic effect if it is given alone, and is always followed by a laxative. In large doses it is cathartic and may produce vertigo, dimness of vision, dilated pupils, muscular spasm, and increased action of the heart.

Spirits

Alcoholic or hydroalcoholic solutions of volatile medicinal substances (chiefly volatile oils).

Sponge Bath

The sponge bath is employed extensively in both acute and chronic diseases, being both simple and convenient. Requiring only a small amount of water, it serves to equalize the circulation, relax the capillaries, reduce fever, and produce a feeling of comfort. Additionally, it allows for the bathing of only a specific portion of the body.

The temperature of a sponge bath will vary depending on the condition of the patient. If the patient is in a weakened state of reduced vitality or poor circulation, a quick application of cool or cold water can be had without the necessity of immersing the entire body.

Sprays

Oily (light liquid petrolatum) medicinal solutions to be used in atomizer or nebulizer for nares and throat.

Squaw Weed (See *Blue Cohosh*)

Static Electricity

Static electricity is an intermittent, pulsating current of high voltage and low amperage. It produces muscular contraction, stimulates metabolism, increases glandular activity, and promotes absorption of nutrients. It also raises the blood pressure. Usually the static current machine is equipped with revolving discs and spark gaps, which are altered to make the current greater in volume and voltage. Modifications of the static current mechanism are called by various names, such as blue-pencil discharge, direct spark, static wave, static induced, static insulation, head breeze, and others. The manufacturers of these machines provide information on the proper placement of the electrodes for specific applications. As with all electrical treatments, they are done with medical supervision. (See *Electrotherapy.*)

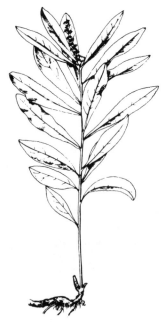

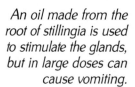

An oil made from the root of stillingia is used to stimulate the glands, but in large doses can cause vomiting.

Stillingia *(Stillingia sylvatica)*

Also known as queen's root or queen's delight, stillingia is native to the southern part of the United States. The root is used as an alterative, an expectorant, a diuretic, a diaphoretic, a sialogogue, a cholagogue, an antivenereal, and in large doses, as an emetic and cathartic. The oil, which is very acrid, is not used internally by itself, as it is a pronounced glandular stimulant. It is often combined with sarsaparilla as a preparation in treating bronchitis, ordinary sore throat, tetter, and syphilis.

The root should be used soon after gathering, since age impairs its effectiveness.

Stomach

Situated between the termination of the esophagus and the beginning of the small intestine, in humans the stomach is the dilated part of the alimentary canal, pyriform in shape and about 12 inches long by 4 inches in diameter.

The mucous membrane of the stomach contains gastric gland openings, through which are secreted pepsin, which acts upon protein, and rennin, which acts upon the casein of milk.

Hydrochloric acid produced in the stomach assists in the breaking down of protein, carbohydrates, and fats, and acts as a powerful stimulant to the intestinal juices. From 8 to 14 pounds of gastric juices are secreted in the stomach every twenty-four hours.

Storax *(Styrax benzoin)*

The balsam obtained from the inner bark of a tree in Asia Minor, also known as styrax. It is used as an expectorant, a stimulant, a mild urinary antiseptic, and, as a local application, as a remedy for scabies. Most often used as a component in the compound tincture of benzoin, it has also been used to treat diphtheria, pulmonic catarrhs, and, when combined with tallow or lard, many forms of skin disease, especially ringworm in children. Since it has a very pleasant taste, it is used in pills; its fragrance is often added to ointments.

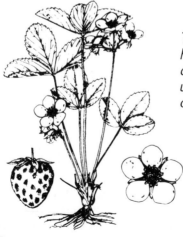

The strawberry plant, highly prized for its delicious fruits, is often used to treat conditions of the skin.

Strawberry

The leaves of the strawberry plant, which is highly prized for its delicious fruit, are used as a mild astringent and diuretic externally in a strong decoction to heal and cleanse eczema and other skin conditions, and internally to aid in the cure of intestinal malfunctions such as diarrhea, dysentery, and affliction of the urinary tract.

A strong tea is made by steeping one teaspoonful of the herb in boiling water for fifteen minutes, or it is often combined with dandelion, burdock, and rhubarb in equal amounts to assure regular bowel evacuation.

The leaves of strawberry as well as the roots and fruit are actively used as a blood purifier and builder. The dose of the tincture is 5 to 15 drops in water three times a day.

Strophanthus Kombé

The sole official use of this East African herb in medicine is for its influence on the circulation, its action being much the same as that of digitalis, the heart-action stimulator.

It is considered highly poisonous when administered without great caution, and is used by the natives to make poison arrowheads. When required in cases of cardiac dropsy, dyspnea, exophthalmos, pulmonary edema, and reflect palpitations of the heart, it is sometimes given hypodermically.

Succus

Vegetable liquids expressed from fresh plants and preserved with alcohol.

Sudorific (See *Diaphoretics*)

Sulphur

A mineral salt naturally present in human blood, its main role is that of helper in the metabolism of proteins. Natural sulphur facilitates sound digestion and the healthy operation of the brain and nervous system, and should be distinguished from "sulfonamide" drugs, which have been found to have bad side effects. Sources of natural sulphur are almonds, Brussels sprouts, cabbage, cauliflower, coconuts, cottage cheese, chestnuts, cranberries, cucumber, red currants, egg yolk, figs, garlic, horseradish, black molasses, okra, onions, oranges, potatoes, pineapple, radishes, and watercress. A large number of herbs also contain natural sulphur in rich quantities. These are: broom tops, calamus, carrageen, coltsfoot, eyebright, fennel seed, meadowseed, mullein, pimpernel, plantain, rest harrow, shepherd's purse, silverweed, stinging nettles, and way-wort.

Sulphur Baths

Sulphur baths are used in the treatment of skin disorders, neuritis, rheumatism, and nervous conditions. The bath solution can be made by dissolving 2 ounces of potassium sulphide in 15 gallons of water, about one-half a tubful. The fluid preparation for a sulphur bath can also be purchased at some pharmacies and used according to the directions.

Sumac *(Rhus glabra)*

A genus of plants of the order of *Anacardiaceae*, of which the sumacs are the best known. *Rhus* is important as a healing agent due to its ability to cause local inflammation by contact with it, thus drawing blood to the area.

Several species of this shrublike plant are found in both Canada and the United States. Care should be taken in their identification, as some are poisonous. The nonpoisonous blue *Glabrum* is easily distinguished by the appearance of its berries in cone-shaped bunches. The sumac leaves are used in a poultice in combination with the crushed fruit for healing of sores, skin ulcers, and wounds.

The bark is used as an astringent and/or a tonic in cases of leucorrhea, rectal difficulties, and chronic diarrhea. It can also be used for all kinds of fevers, cankers in the mouth, and as an astringent gargle for sore throats. A tea made from the berries combined with blueberry is used to treat diabetes. A syrup can be made by covering the berries with boiling water, steeping for one hour, then straining, and adding honey; in this form it can be easily stored.

Sumbul (Musk root) *Ferula sumbul*

The root is distinguished by its musklike odor and bitter taste. It is used as a nerve tonic and as a substitute for musk. Mainly found in Turkey, Russia, and northern India, it is used as a stimulant, an antispasmodic, and to treat various hysterical conditions. It is widely used in dysmenorrhea and allied female disorders because of its specific action on the pelvic organs. Sumbul is also employed in chronic dysentery and diarrhea, as well as in chronic bronchitis, especially with asthmatic conditions and pneumonia.

The recognized source of sumbul in the United States is false sumbul, the root of the *Dorema ammoniacum.*

Suppository

A solid, medicated compound designed for insertion into the rectum, urethra, or vagina. It is specifically composed to retain its shape while at room temperature and to melt at the temperature of the human body. The basis of most suppositories is oil of theobroma, with the exception of the urethral suppositories, which are made with a mixture of gelatin and glycerin.

Rectal suppositories should be cone- or spindle-shaped and should weigh about 2 grams. Vaginal suppositories should be globular or oviform in shape and weigh about 10 grams if made with gelatin and about 4 grams if made with oil of theobroma.

Suppositories for use in the urethra should be pencil-shaped and pointed at one end and should weigh 2 grams if approximately 7 centimeters in length, and 4 grams if 14 centimeters in length. If urethral suppositories use oil of theobroma as a base, they should weigh about one-half of the above.

Suppuration

The production of pus, or suppuration, is nearly always due to the presence of bacteria such as the streptococcus, the staphylococcus, the gonococcus, or the bacillus pyocyaneus. Pus is a thick, creamy, opaque, yellowish white fluid having a faint odor and salty taste. Collections of pus are called abscesses and can be either superficial and acute or chronic and deep-seated.

Acute suppuration is accompanied by marked inflammatory symptoms such as swelling, changes in the surrounding skin, and throbbing pain. Chronic abscesses are often present without inflammatory symptoms and are thought to be produced by the tubercle bacillus.

Abscesses or suppuration are treated most often by early incision under strict antiseptic conditions. The abscess cavity is scraped and cleansed, and drainage is introduced, followed by the application of antiseptic dressings.

As systemic disturbances in the body can occur in the presence of suppuration, tonics, stimulants, anodynes, and nutritious foods are employed to repair damage to the body.

Sweat Baths

The underlying principle of the many kinds of sweat baths is producing perspiration to cleanse the body of its large quantities of effete or waste matter. The sweat bath is used to relieve internal congestion, equalize circulation, stimulate glandular and cellular activity, stimulate the nervous system, and aid in the digestive processes of the body. Patients with rheumatism, catarrh, neuritis, auto intoxication, nervousness, chronic inflammations, kidney diseases, and afflictions of the skin are often given sweat baths.

The most widely used and suitable cabinet for giving the sweat bath is the hot-air cabinet, which delivers dry heat by means of electric lights. Patients can be placed in either the upright or reclining cabinet, the latter one being desirable for patients who suffer from weak heart actions, making it possible for them to lie down.

Sweat baths are generally taken no more often than three times weekly and at least two hours after any meal. When a patient has begun to perspire freely, it is indicated that he or she has been in the cabinet long enough. If symptoms of restlessness, rapid heartbeat, discomfort, or depression occur, the bath should be discontinued immediately. The amount of time that individuals can remain comfortably in the cabinet depends upon their general body condition, but the average length of most sweat baths is somewhere between ten and twenty-five minutes.

A towel wrung out of cold water can be placed around the patient's head and neck to prevent the possibility of fainting during the bath, and the presence of someone in the room during the patient's stay in the cabinet is extremely desirable. Upon removal of the patient from the cabinet, it is often wise to open the cabinet door first, to allow the temperature change to become more gradual for the patient.

Quicker and more profuse perspiration during a sweat bath can be aided by giving the patient a glass of hot water or hot lemonade prior to the bath. After the bath, the patient can be given a sponge or shower bath to remove the perspiration from the body, and some practitioners follow the bath with a massage or some manipulative movements of the body.

Caution should be exercised in giving sweat baths to patients with diseases of heart weakness, high blood pressure, or lowered vitality or any kind. (See also *Hot-Air Treatments.*)

Syrups

Concentrated solutions of sucrose, the menstruum being an aqueous solution of either medicinal or flavoring agents (simple syrup menstruum—distilled water). A *cordial* is a one-fourth-weaker medicated syrup.

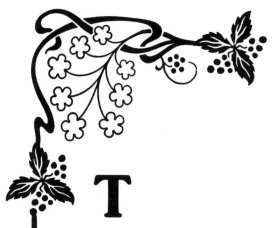

T

Tampon

Generally constructed of sterile cotton gauze, the most common tampons are used to absorb menstrual blood flow from the uterus, being designed to fit comfortably in the vaginal canal. Tampons used for the purpose of medicating pelvic and uterine inflammatory conditions are often made of lamb's wool and saturated with glycerin or a 10-percent solution of ichthyol and glycerin. Used for this purpose, the tampons are usually removed after twenty-four hours and followed by a hot vaginal douche.

Tampons are used effectively to apply continued pressure in backward displacements of the uterus complicated by slight adhesions, and are usually renewed daily.

Tannic Acid

The principal use of this drug is as an astringent application to mucous membranes. It is a solid, uncrystallizable, glucoside obtained from vegetable astringents, and is very soluble in water and glycerin. The most common preparations of the substance are ointments, troches, and styptic collodions.

Tannic acid is incompatible with the alkaloids such as iron or albumin. Most black teas contain tannic acid.

Tapotement

A form of muscle treatment or massage administered by rapid strikes to the body with the hands or fingers. It is excellent in treating atrophied conditions of the muscles, as it increases contraction of the muscle fiber, increases blood supply, stimulates the nerves, and generally hardens the muscle.

Blows are given from the wrist and are short and quick, with four varying percussions: hacking—striking with the ulnar border of the hand to muscle and around the nerve centers; tapping—striking with the tips of the fingers, chiefly around the heart and upon the head; clapping—striking with the palms or flat surface of the hands and fingers, on the superficial nerves and vessels of the skin (cupping the hand varies this movement slightly); and beating—striking with the ulnar surface of the closed hand, on the buttocks and lower extremities, over the sciatic nerve.

Tea (*Camellia thea*)

The term has come to be used broadly to describe a beverage, usually hot, made from boiling various herbs or other ingredients in mixtures together in water. There are literally thousands of "teas" on the market today, containing almost every known spice and flavor. In medical discussion, the term is widely used to describe the dosage form that is most often drunk.

Specifically, tea or *Thea,* the leaves of the *Camellia thea,* a Chinese evergreen shrub, contains an alkaloid the action of which is identical with that of caffeine, found in coffee. Black and green tea are both prepared from the same plant, the difference lying in the length of time the leaves are exposed to air and the number of times they are roasted and rolled, the green being less treated.

Tea is used medicinally as an astringent and a stimulant, exerting a definite influence over the nervous system and usually producing a feeling of comfort and exhilaration. Taken in large quantity, however, it causes unnatural wakefulness and will produce unpleasant nervous and dyspeptic symptoms. The green variety appears to have the greatest effect on the nerves.

Teeth

Embedded in the alveolar process of the jaw bones, the teeth, which are necessary organs of digestion, first appear in temporary form in infants about six to seven months old.

The teeth are shaped and located in the jaw structure according to their function in the processing of consumed food.

The first set of teeth, or milk teeth, numbers twenty (10 upper and 10 lower), and the second or permanent set numbers thirty two (16 upper and 16 lower). Both sets of teeth are composed of incisors for cutting; canines, also for cutting; bicuspids (premolars) for grinding; and molars for grinding.

Temperature

The normal temperature of the body in a state of health is 98.6° F, when measured in the mouth. Measured in the vagina or rectum, it is 0.3 to 0.6° F higher. The body temperature is lowest between two and six A.M. and reaches its highest normal temperature between five and eight P.M. Almost any disturbance of the equilibrium in the body can result in raising or lowering the temperature.

Temperature Diagnosis

The accurate and frequent recording of the temperature is a widely used method of determining disturbance in the body. A higher than normal temperature is indicative of fever, the body's own mechanism for fighting off alien organisms. There is also evidence that temperatures can rise in the presence of emotional disturbances. Body temperature below normal can be caused by blood loss, diabetes, exposure, myxedema, or peritonitis.

Testicles

The glandular organs of the male in which semen is produced and from which it is secreted. Two oval bodies also called the testes, they are suspended in the scrotum by the spermatic cord. Each testicle weighs from ¾ to 1 ounce.

In the fetus, the testes are located in the abdominal cavity, just below the kidneys. Descent into the scrotum begins in about the fifth and is usually complete in the eighth month of gestation.

Thorn Apple *(Datura stramonium)*

The leaves of this coarse plant are used medicinally. Containing the same alkaloids as belladonna, but in smaller proportion, it is used as an antispasmodic, an anodyne, and an antinarcotic, as is belladonna, but is considered slightly more sedative than the latter.

Also called stramonium, in the East Indies this herb has been employed to treat conditions of spasmodic asthma; it is smoked or burned as a powder to be inhaled. The beneficial effect is believed to be due to the presence of atropine, which paralyzes the ends of the pulmonary branches, thereby relieving the spasm.

Applied locally as ointments, plasters, or fomentations, it is used to alleviate the pain of muscular rheumatism, neuralgia, hemorrhoids, fistulae, and abscesses.

Thyme *(Thymus vulgaris)*

An herb recognized around the world for flavoring as well as for ornamental decor, garden thyme has a strong, pungent, spicy taste and odor. The herb is collected in the summer, when its pale lilac flowers are in bloom, and thoroughly dried in the shade.

Thyme is used medicinally as a tonic, a carminative, an emmenagogue, and an antispasmodic. An infusion of 1 teaspoonful to 1 cup of boiling water, steeped for ½ hour, is taken; or of the tincture, 20 to 50 drops in hot water.

Externally, the oil of thyme is used for toothache, neuralgia, and painful swellings.

Thyroid Gland

A gland surrounding the front and sides of the upper part of the trachea and the lower sides of the larynx, its function is to secrete thyroxin, which aids in the metabolism process in the body.

The thyroid gland is encapsulated in two layers, and consists of a right and left lobe. Myxedema and mental failures are attributed to the loss or degeneration of thyroid, and cretinism to the arrest in the gland's development.

Thyroxin

The active principle of the thyroid gland, it contains 63 percent iodine. Dosage medicinally is usually 1/120 grain, given in the event of removal or failure of the thyroid gland.

Tibb-i Unaani

Tibb-i Unaani (literally, "Medicine of the Greeks") may be defined as that system of Greek medicine which has been developed by Muslim civilization. Muslims call it Tibb-i Unaani in India, Pakistan, and Afghanistan, acknowledging its Ionian origin, whereas European historians call it Arab or Islamic medicine. At present, at the largest institute in the world for study of and teaching of the Tibb system (Hamdard Foundation at New Delhi, India), it is now referred to as Tibb-i Islami, perhaps the most correct of all the various terminology.

This system of medicine is based on the Pythagorean theory of the four primary qualities—hot, cold, wet, and dry—of the elements (Earth, Water, Air, and Fire) and the Hippocratic humoral theory. The theory supposes the presence in the body of four humours (in Arabic, *Akhlat*): blood, phlegm, yellow bile, and black bile. The temperaments of persons are accordingly expressed by the words *sanguine, phlegmatic, choleric,* and *melancolic,* according to the preponderance in them of one of the humours.

The humours themselves are given temperaments: blood is hot and moist, phlegm, cold and moist; yellow bile, hot and dry; and black bile, cold and dry. Plant and mineral substances are also assigned temperaments, and there are degrees of these temperaments.

Every person is felt to have a unique humoral constitution, which represents his or her healthy state. Any change in the humours brings about a change in the state of health. There is formulated also a power of self-preservation or adjustment, which strives to restore any disturbance within the limits prescribed by the constitution or state of the individual. This corresponds to the "defense mechanism," which is employed in case of insult to the body.

Practitioners of the Tibb system are called *hakims* (feminine: *hakima*), and the mode of analysis of a patient's condition is to consider first all aspects of the person's life—one's will, desires, inclination, nature, habits, and customs. The total person is examined in respect to general virility, weight, mental and physical state, digestive capacity, condition of the intestines and humours, the weather, climate, the environment, eating habits, occupation, mode of living, and so forth. Frequently, diagnosis of the specific imbalance of a humour is determined in a matter of seconds by resorting to pulse diagnosis.

Recipes/prescriptions in the Tibb system are comprised of natural herbal substances and some animal and mineral substances, based upon the temperament (hot/cold/moist/dry) of the person and the synergistic effect of the compounded herbs. The object of such a treatment is not to treat any specific disease but to reform the whole external and internal biotic environment.

Every imbalance is observed in the Tibb system to pass through three stages, culminating in the healing crisis. The first stage, acridity, is the time of irritation, cause, or the initial state; the second phase is the time of ripening, when the actual crisis may occur; the third stage is solution, resulting in either cure or death. The day in which the crisis occurs, various signs usually occur that signal the innate healing system of the body and act to expel superfluous morbid matter in the form of nosebleeding, sweating, urination, diarrhea, or vomiting. Critical days usually occur in four- and seven-day cycles (or multiples of these numbers). For a complete cure to occur, it is felt that the crisis must occur in one of these five forms, and furthermore, that the affected morbid humour must be ripened or "thickened" prior to expulsion.

While the origins of the Tibb system are clearly acknowledged to be in the ancient Greek and specifically Hippocratic philosophy, practically speaking, the single most influential figure in the Unaani Tibb system was Hakim Ibn Sina (Avicenna). *The Canon of Medicine,* his chief medical work, is a codifying and ordering of all medical knowledge that existed in the world up to his time. In eighteen volumes, it maintained its authority through seven centuries of medical teaching and practice, and today remains the sourcebook and *materia medica* for the *hakims*. (See also *Avicenna, Arab Medicine.*)

Tinctures

Vinegar, alcoholic, or hydroalcoholic solutions of nonvolatile herb constituents. To make tinctures of fresh drugs, put 50 teaspoons of fresh herb, cut, bruised or crushed, for 15 days, in a stoppered container with 75 cubic centimeters alcohol, or vinegar, agitating several times per day. Drain onto filter, through which add alcohol or vinegar to make 100 centimeters.

Tissue

Body tissue is comprised of a group of *like* cells performing a particular function; fine basic tissue groups working together comprise an *organ,* and several organs connected for performing highly specialized functions are called a *system.*

     Epithelial tissue—covers the entire surface of the body; its function is that of protection and secretion. The epithelial cells in the skin are the epidermi, reproduced as quickly as they are destroyed by friction. They continuously protect the blood vessels and nerves from injury. In the digestive tract and glands, epithelial tissue secretes a digestion-aiding fluid; in the nose, throat, and lungs, it serves a lubricatory function.

     Connective tissue—found throughout the body, this tissue makes up the supporting, binding, and connecting parts of other cells. It forms the foundation for all organs, nerves, and blood vessels.

     Muscle tissue—provides the power of contraction for the body, both voluntary and involuntary.

     Vascular tissue—conveys materials to the body parts, for example, lymph and blood tissue.

     Nervous tissue—conducts nerve impulses to the various body parts.

Tobacco

The dried leaves of a native American plant containing nicotine, which is an emetic, a depressant, an antispasmodic, and a diaphoretic. Used occasionally for medical purposes, nicotine is a rapidly paralyzing poison in large quantities.

Tonics

Agents that are taken usually to promote nutrition and tone the system. Certain tonics act especially on specific areas of the body and are given in varying forms such as pills, tinctures, and simple syrups.

Strychnine is given to patients requiring treatment of poor circulation and of disorders based in the spinal cord. For their effect on the heart and its disorders, digitalis, squill, convallarin, and cirricifuga are given as tonics, and for the nerve system, phosphorous and quinine.

Toxicology

The study of the effect, nature, and detection of drugs when given in poisonous doses, as well as the treatment and antidotes for same.

Trace Element Therapy

George H. Earp-Thomas of Bloomfield Labs in New Jersey found that he could cure a very high percentage of cancer patients by supplying the mineral salts which were deficient in the patient's body, as determined by blood tests.

He was successful in isolating and photographing three forms of the cancer germ and is said never to have lost a case with those patients where a blood test showed either of two forms of the germ present (90 percent of all cases). In the remaining 10 percent of the cases (where the third form was present), only the pain could be relieved. Thousands of patients are said to have been cured from 1900 to 1948 by this method at a Richmond, Virginia, hospital.

Other researchers are convinced that every one of the ninety-two naturally occurring chemical elements ("minerals") are necessary for the body. At least one manufacturer sells tablets containing all ninety-two minerals in natural form.

Triticum *(Agrophyon repens)*

Although it is known widely as couch grass and generally regarded as a worthless, prolific, and troublesome weed, its roots are nevertheless considered a valuable source of food by knowledgable farmers of cattle and horses. The roots, having a sweet taste somewhat resembling that of licorice, have been marketed in Europe and used there for grinding into meal to make bread.

Historically, roots of couch grass have been used as a springtime tonic to purify blood, and in cases of urinary stones in the bladder. Even today, couch grass as a diuretic and demulcent is used often in the treatment for cystitis and catarrhal diseases of the bladder. For rheumatism and gout, an infusion is made using 1 ounce of the dried crushed root in 1 pint of boiling water. Its diuretic effect is apparently owing to the sugar content.

Troches

Solid, round, oval, or flat masses of one or more medicinal agents, with sucrose or extract of glycorrhiza, or both, caused to adhere by tragacanth mucilage, often flavored. Also called lozenges, tablets. In England, of definite weight and chocolate base.

Turkish Bath

A dry hot-air treatment ranging from 145 to 200°F, usually lasting from 10 to 25 minutes, depending on the patient's stamina, and most often followed by exposure to gradually cooler steam and a shower to remove the perspiration. The patient is then massaged for 15 to 20 minutes and given two more showers—first hot or warm and then cold water.

Turpentine

Containing a volatile oil which is stimulant, antispasmodic, diuretic, and anthelmintic, turpentine is derived from several species of pine trees.

Externally, turpentine is used as a rubefacient, having a powerful effect on the skin. The dose of the oil taken internally is 5 to 15 drops; of the oleoresin, 5 to 31 grains. (See also *Cajuput Oil.*)

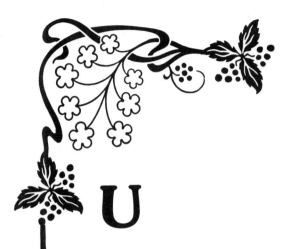

U

Ultraviolet Rays (See *Finsen Light*)

Uric Acid

The small quantity of acid that is found in the urine. An increase of uric acid (excretion of over 1 gram) is found where there is excessive tissue waste, acute rheumatic fever, renal or vesical stones, and when there is an excessive use of protein foods and particularly coffee. A decrease (excretion of less than ¼ gram) is found in diminished tissue waste, kidney diseases, vegetarian diet, or diminished protein diet, particularly those foods free from purine bases. (A purine base is one of the waste-products of normal biochemical bodily function with an especially acidic quality. Caffeine and uric acid are two examples.)

Urinalysis

An examination of the secretions of the kidneys used in the diagnosis of disease. To be complete, urinalysis must include examination physically, chemically, and microscopically. Diabetes and Bright's disease are the two principal diseases in which the examination furnishes positive and reliable evidence through the disclosure of sugar and albumin in the urine.

Urine is formed by the action of the kidneys in removing waste material from the blood. The filtering and secretion of the kidneys form the urine, which is conveyed by drops into the bladder, which distends and holds approximately 1 pint. Few practitioners have the time or facilities for making a complete examination of the urine. Therefore, it is the usual practice, when such examination is needed, to send the sample to a laboratory or to an analytical chemist.

Tests for albumin and sugar content may be done at home. In testing for albumin content, a small amount of urine is placedcin a clean glass tube and slowly brought to a boil over a small flame. If albumin is present, it will coagulate or clump together like the white of an egg. The test for sugar content is done with the aid of Fehling's or Haine's solution which is available at most drugstores. Into a clean tube place 25 to 30 drops of one of the aforementioned solutions. Freshness is assured if the solution remains deep blue when it is brought to a boil. Then add 10 to 15 drops of urine and bring to a boil again. If sugar is present, an abundant yellow or brick red dust color is present. If sugar is absent, no change should take place.

Acidity of the urine may be tested by dipping blue litmus paper into the urine. If the paper turns red, the reaction is acid. If there is no change when the blue paper is used, dip a piece of red litmus paper in the same manner and if it turns blue, the urine is alkaline. Should there be no change in either paper, the condition is neutral. The urine is normally acid in reaction. "Nitrazine" paper is often used to test pH of urine. Noting the amount, color, and odor of the secretion is often useful in diagnosis. In a twenty-four-hour period, a healthy man normally passes approximately 50 ounces of urine. An increase may be due to diabetes, chronic interstitial nephritis, high blood pressure, dropsical affusions, or some nervous disorders such as hysteria. A decrease may be due to fever, low blood pressure, diarrhea, cholera, or acute or chronic parenchymatous nephritis.

The normal color of the urine is pale yellow. When there is diabetes, it becomes very pale, even colorless. If it is brownish or reddish, there is blood in the urine. If a minute amount of blood is present, it may be smokelike in color. Orange color may be an indication of fever or jaundice, or only excessively hard work. Very yellow urine indicates presence of bile and probable liver disorders. Opalescent urine contains microorganisms, and whitish or milky urine indicates chyle fats or pus.

Bluish urine may be due to typhus or poisoning from methylene; blue and greenish urine comes from heavy bile, creosote, or coal tar in the system. Blackish urine indicates overdoses of coal-tar derivatives or guaiacol creosote, and liver disorders. The odor is also informative. Normally the odor of urine is remarkable and slightly sharp to the nose, intensifying if there is any acetone present. It smells unpleasantly like ammonia if it is decomposing. Urine may smell like fresh violets if the patient has been absorbing turpentine. Persistent scalding symptoms during urination should be attended to at once, since this is sometimes a sign of gonorrhea.

Uterus

The uterus is a hollow, pear-shaped, muscular organ measuring about 3 inches long, 2 inches broad, and 1 inch thick, flattened from the front backward. It is placed base upward, forming an angle with the vagina, which par-

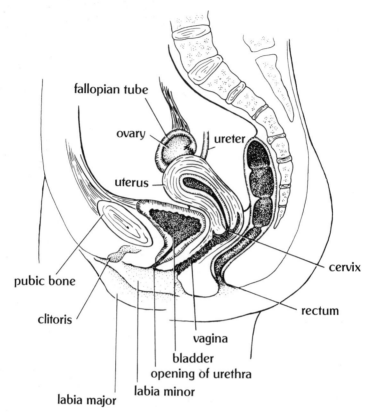

Female Reproductive Organs

tially receives the cervix. The uterus is situated in the pelvic cavity, between the bladder in front and the rectum behind.

Uva-ursi (See *Bearberry*)

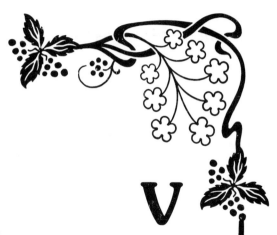

Valerian (*Valeriana officinalis*)

The rhizome and rootlets of *Valeriana officinalis,* it is used as an antispasmodic and a stimulant and is of value in treatment of hysteria, convulsions due to worms, coma of typhus fever, and whooping cough. The must used preparation is a solvent in water; its bodily influence is antispasmodic, calmative, stimulating, tonic, and nervine.

Valerian is used by herbalists today primarily as a nerve tonic and is often combined with skullcap, blue vervain, mistletoe, gentian, or peppermint, which increases the promptness of its action. It is also employed in the treatment of St. Vitus's dance (chorea), nervous derangement or irritations, debility, hysterical afflictions (especially female), and wakefulness during fever. In large doses, it has been known to cause headaches, mental excitement, hallucinations, giddiness, restlessness, agitation, and even spasmodic movement. Normal dosage is ½ teaspoon of the tincture, a wineglass of the infusion, 3 to 5 grains of the extract, or 5 drops of the oil. Externally, an infusion of ½ cup of the root may be used in a bath to relieve nervous exhaustion. Valerian has an odor peculiarly obnoxious to humans, but cats seem to prefer valerian to catnip.

Vermifuge (See *Anthelmintic*)

Vibration

Vibration is performed by placing the hand or fingers upon the body and rapidly shaking by trembling, pressing movements. The vibrating hand should occasionally be moved. Such action increases the contractile power of muscles and is also of value in the treatment of neuritis and neuralgia after the inflammatory stage is past.

Vibration is also a powerful means of stimulating the circulation, glandular activity, and nervous plexi, and also acts as a stimulus to the peristaltic movement of the intestines. The exercise should take approximately five minutes.

There are several models of mechanical vibrators on the market which require the use of electricity for operation and often give excellent satisfaction for vibratory massage. This procedure should not be used in skin afflictions, burns, sores, tumors, purulent inflammation, fevers, serious diseases of the circulatory system, blood diseases, inflamed joints, or during pregnancy, menstruation (although sometimes ordered in treatment for scanty or retarded flow), acute bone diseases, and all conditions in which there is a possible danger of producing hemorrhage.

Violet *(Viola odorata)*

The leaves and flowers, which are solvent in boiling water, are the medicinal part of violet, which is found throughout North America. The influence of the dissolving properties seems to have an intricate ability to reach places only the blood and lymphatic fluids penetrate. It is used for treatment of difficult breathing and when gas, distension, and pressure are caused by a morbid accumulation of material in the stomach and bowels.

Violet tea taken daily for some time is cooling to any high temperature of the body. It is of value in the treatment of headaches. Violet is a specific treatment for ear disturbances, since it has a soothing and healing effect on inflamed mucous surfaces. Problems such as colds, sore throat, inflammation of lungs, hoarseness, and whooping cough, in children and adults, are greatly controlled by a handful of dried or fresh violet leaves and flowers in ½ pint of water steeped for a half-hour. Administer 2 to 3 tablespoons (more for adults) every two to three hours, or give a mouthful as a gargle. (Make sure the bowels eliminate properly.) As a tea, use 1 teaspoon of the herb to 1 cup of boiling water. Externally, crushed violet leaves are bound as a compress on inflamed tumors, sore throats, swollen breasts, and to the back of the head and neck for headache. A cloth saturated in violet tea will often give good results if it is applied for an extended period.

Violet Ray

A vacuum electrode of high-frequency current often produces a violet color in a glass tube, which led to the coining of the term ultraviolet rays, although there are no true ultraviolet rays produced by this method. The violet-ray treatment provides a bathing of the parts with ozone, a refined form of oxygen which results from a break in the electrical current. During this treatment, large quantities of ozone are driven into the cells of the body, and the body retains the characteristic odor of ozone for many hours after the treatment.

Vitamins

Vitamins are important food elements that are absolutely necessary for the normal maintenance of good health. While vitamins may not be building materials, they are essential to enable the body to utilize these materials. Five vitamins were originally isolated and named. Since then, many more have been added to the list.

Like organic salts and minerals, vitamins are found in the vegetable kingdom, in fruits, and in natural or unrefined foods. In modern commercial processes of refining or chemically treating foods, vitamins are often lost or changed so drastically as to render them useless. A deficiency of vitamins and lack of mineral salts may result in general weakness and be the cause of many chronic and lingering diseases. The absence of these substances in the diet leads to functional and degenerative changes in the central nervous system and to similar changes in every organ and tissue in the body.

The complex symptoms resulting from the absence of vitamin substances are mineral starvation, derangements of the functions of the organs of digestion, disordered endocrine function, and malnutrition of the nervous system.

Certain organs of the body atrophy or diminish in size when vitamins are lacking in the system. These organs include: testicles, spleen, ovaries, pancreas, heart, liver, kidneys, stomach, thyroid, and brain.

Gastric, intestinal, biliary, and pancreatic insufficiency are important consequences of a diet too rich in starch and too poor in vitamins and other essential constituents of food. Vitamin deficiency also has a noticeable effect on the organs of reproduction, in both the male and female, frequently resulting in sterility. The efficiency of vitamins is greatly impaired or destroyed by excessive heat. Canned foods are therefore deficient in vitamins as well as other mineral elements and should never constitute a large part of one's diet. (See also listings for individual vitamins A, B, C, D, E, K, and appendices.)

Vomiting

Solid food ejected from the stomach in certain forms of dyspepsia and after the ingestion of partly decomposed food may be produced by a variety of local and reflex causes, and also during infectious fevers. *Acid vomiting* is dyspepsia with hyperacidity and constipation. *Mucous vomiting* is a symptom of acute and chronic gastritis. Bile is present in the vomitus, in obstruction of the bowels in the early stages, in the impaction of a gallstone, and in malarial or yellow fever. Fecal vomiting is a symptom of the later stages of intestinal obstruction. *Hematemesis,* or vomiting of blood, is seen in gastric cancer, ulceration of the stomach, yellow fever, and sometimes in cirrhosis of the liver. Rupture of an abscess in the stomach or esophagus will produce purulent vomiting.

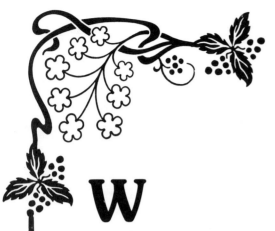

W

Wahoo *(Euonymus europaeus)*

The bark of *Euonymus europaeus* is an astringent, tonic and a purgative, resembling in action such plants as rhubarb, jalap, and aloe, but it is milder. The extract is given in doses of 1 to 5 grains for dropsy and hepatic afflictions. Up to 3 grains are given as a tonic, laxative and purgative.

Waste, Bodily

The waste products of the body consist of urea, carbon dioxide, salt, and water. They leave the body by way of the lungs, kidneys, and skin, which are the three principal channels of elimination. The bowels eliminate a small amount of waste substances; their chief function, however, is to discharge the undigested portion of food. (See also *Large Intestine*.)

Water

Potable water is fit for humans to drink. Unpotable water is not. Good drinking water should be clear and limpid, colorless, odorless, free of sulphurated hydrogen or putrefied animal matter; it should not be too cold, but should have a temperature of 46 to 60° F; it should have an agreeable taste—neither flat, nor salty, nor sweetish; it should be as free as possible of dissolved organic matter, especially of animal origin; it should not contain over 3 or 4 parts of chlorine in 100,000 parts of water. Diseases that may be transmitted in drinking water include: typhoid, cholera, dysentery, diarrhea, vesical calculi, intestinal worms, and lead poisoning.

Wax Ceratum

Ointment made firmer by the addition of wax; softens but does not melt at body temperature, and liquefies only above 40° C (104° F).

Weight

Body weight is a valuable means of determining the state of metabolism. Maintaining one's correct weight is important for good health. The weight, to a certain extent, shows the condition of the nutritive and assimilative powers of the individual. Medical examiners lay great stress upon body weight and insist that the weight of all applicants to the armed forces and all those applying for life insurance fall within the standard range.

Desirable Weights for Men and Women
(According to height and frame, age 25 and over)

Height		Weight (lb) in Indoor Clothing[a]		
Ft.	In.	Small Frame	Medium Frame	Large Frame
(in shoes, 1-in. heels)			*Men*	
5	2	112–120	118–129	126–141
5	3	115–123	121–133	129–144
5	4	118–126	124–136	132–148
5	5	121–129	127–139	135–152
5	6	124–133	130–143	138–156
5	7	128–137	134–147	142–161
5	8	132–141	138–152	147–166
5	9	136–145	142–156	151–170
5	10	140–150	146–160	155–174
5	11	144–154	150–165	159–179
6	0	148–158	154–170	164–184
6	1	152–162	158–175	168–189
6	2	156–167	162–180	173–194
6	3	160–171	167–185	178–199
6	4	164–175	172–190	182–204
(in shoes, 2-in. heels)			*Women*	
4	10	92– 98	96–107	104–119
4	11	94–101	98–110	106–122
5	0	96–104	101–113	109–125
5	1	99–107	104–116	112–128
5	2	102–110	107–119	115–131
5	3	105–113	110–122	118–134
5	4	108–116	113–126	121–138
5	5	111–119	116–130	125–142
5	6	114–123	120–135	129–146
5	7	118–127	124–139	133–150

5	8	122–131	128–143	137–154
5	9	126–135	132–147	141–158
5	10	130–140	136–151	145–163
5	11	134–144	140–155	149–168
6	0	138–148	144–159	153–173

[a]SOURCE: The Metropolitan Life Insurance Company. Derived primarily from data of the Build and Blood Pressure Study, 1959, Society of Actuaries.

Wheatgrass Manna

A method for treating cancer, leukemia, and many other ailments is drinking freshly prepared juice of wheat grass. This therapy can be used in conjunction with other treatments.

The method of preparation, developed by Ann Wigmore, D.D., 25 Exeter Street, Boston, Massachusetts, 02116, appears in the booklet *Wheatgrass— God's Manna,* issued by the National Medical-Physical Research Foundation, Inc.

Taken with a simple diet (consisting mainly of fresh raw fruits and vegetables), wheat grass juice betters the health.

The book *Why Suffer?* by Ann Wigmore (privately circulated) gives natural living and healing instructions, based on actual experience, combined with what she has learned about wheat grass manna.

White Pine *(Pinus Strobus)*

The medicinal parts are the inner bark or sprigs, which are solvent in boiling water. White pine is an expectorant. The resin is used for the treatment of colds, rheumatism, tuberculosis, influenza, chronic indigestion, and kidney trouble. The bark and new sprigs are useful in modifying the quality and quantity of the mucous secretions and to bring about their removal in bronchial and catarrhal trouble, rheumatism, scurvy, all chest infections, tonsillitis, laryngitis, croup, and the like. The dosage is the combination of 1 teaspoonful each of the following with 1 pint of water: white pine, wild cherry bark, sassafras, and spikenard. Steep the mixture for a half-hour and administer a half-teaspoonful to a mouthful every hour, depending on age and condition of the patient. It is further of use with bearberry, marshmallow, and poplar bark for the treatment of diabetes. The dosage of the above preparation is three to 4 cupfuls daily, and if the tincture is used, ½ to 1 fluid dram.

Used externally, the heated resin of white pine is a dressing which draws out imbedded splinters or brings boils to a head. Sores, cuts, swellings, and insect bites also repond favorably to this treatment. The hot resin may also be spread on a warm cloth and applied as one would a mustard plaster for the treatment of pneumonia, sciatic pain, and any general muscular soreness.

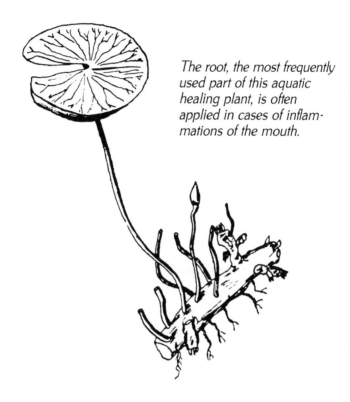

The root, the most frequently used part of this aquatic healing plant, is often applied in cases of inflammations of the mouth.

White Pond Lily *(Nymphaea odorata)*

The root of the white pond lily, soluble in water, is the medicinal part of the plant. It is primarily antiseptic, astringent, demulcent, and discutient. The infusion is healing to sores, ulcerated mouth, inflamed gums, canker, and sore throat. Tincture of the root is useful in treatment of back pain, coryza, diarrhea, and sore throat. The dosage is 1 ounce of the root boiled in 1 pint of water for twenty minutes, taken in amounts of a wineglassful to a teacupful two or three times a day. The fluidextract dosage is 10 to 15 drops morning and night. Externally, the fresh juice of the root mixed with lemon juice is excellent for removing freckles, pimples, and dark discolorations of the skin. Made into a strong tea, white pond lily is useful in the treatment of painful swelling, boils, ulcers, and the like when applied with cotton or towels. The bruised leaves are healing to wounds and cuts when they are applied as a poultice.

Wintergreen *(Gaultheria procumbens)*

The leaf of the American evergreen plant, *Gaultheria procumbens,* is used to extract the volatile oil and spirit. The oil is composed of about 90 percent methyl salicylate. Its physiological action is useful in rheumatism and gout, in doses of 3 to 10 minims, in capsule form or dropped onto sugar. Externally, it is used in many liniments.

Witch Hazel *(Hamamelis virginiana)*

A tea made of the leaves is excellent for many complaints such as bleeding of the stomach, which can be treated either by chewing the leaves or drinking a tea. It is also serviceable in treatment of complaints of the bowels, piles, and complaints common to females. In bearing-down pains of labor, it gives relief if properly administered.

Wormwood *(Artemisia absinthium)*

The tops and leaves are used as a tonic, a stomachic, a stimulant febrifuge, an anthelmintic, and a narcotic. Soluble in alcohol and partially in water, it is first-rate in treatment of enfeebled digestion and debility.

Often melancholy is due to liver inactivity, and a small amount of wormwood given daily will decrease the yellowness of the skin, revealing improvement of the gall bladder. It is also used for the treatment of intermittent fever, jaundice, loss of appetite, amenorrhea, chronic leucorrhea, diabetes, obstinate diarrhea, swelling of the tonsils, and quinsy. If the dosage is too strong or if it is given too often, it will irritate the stomach. The dosage is 1 teaspoon of the tops and leaves, cut small or granulated, to 1 cup of boiling water taken in wineglassfuls three or four times a day. Of the tincture, 5 to 30 drops three or four times daily (according to age and condition). Oil of wormwood is an effective ingredient in liniment for sprains, bruises, lumbago, and so on. Tincture of the fresh root is used to expel worms.

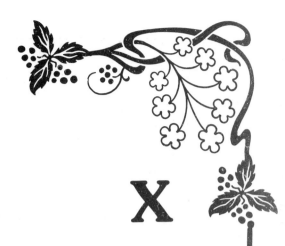

Xanthine

An alkaloid found in nearly all the tissues and liquids of living animals and in many plants, xanthine is also found in minute quantities as a normal constituent of the urine. It is formed by decomposition of nuclein by dilute acids. Xanthine is probably oxidized in the body as fast as it is formed. It is a colorless powder, almost insoluble in cold water but readily soluble in dilute acids and alkalies. It is nonpoisonous and is a muscle stimulant, especially to the heart.

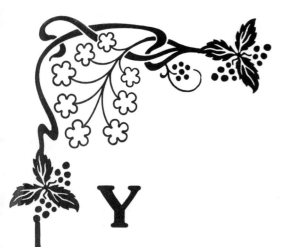

Y

Yarrow *(Achillea millefolium)*

Yarrow is used as an astringent, an alterative, a diuretic, and a tonic. Herbalists use yarrow to stop hemorrhages of the lungs, bowels, hemorrhoids, and other internal bleeding. It is most useful in the treatment of colds, influenza, measles, smallpox, chickenpox, fevers, and acute catarrhs of the respiratory tract.

Yarrow acts as a blood cleanser and opens the pores to permit free perspiration, taking along with it unwanted waste and thus relieving the kidneys. Yarrow exercises influence over many ailments, including incontinence of the urine and mucous discharges from the bladder, dyspepsia, amenorrhea (suppressed menses), and in menorrhagia (profuse, continued menstruation). It is also used in solution for leucorrhea. Internal decoction of yarrow boiled with white wine is used to slow menstrual discharge. Chewing the leaves will frequently ease the pain of toothache.

Yawning

This may be due to indigestion, fatigue, or lack of ventilation, or it may be imitative. It is characterized by a deep inspiration, sudden depression of the lower jaw, a clicking sound, stretching of the limbs, and a prolonged expiration, accompanied by a loud sound. It is confined to the area controlled by the fifth cranial nerve.

Yellow Dock *(Rumex crispus)*

The root of this plant is often made into an ointment to ease itching. The roots should be bruised fine in a mortar and enough cream added to make an ointment. Keep the mixture warm for twelve hours, taking care not to scald it. Rub it on at night before retiring. Three applications are usually enough to effect a cure. This ointment together with lobelia and a few drops of spirit of turpentine will be sufficient to cure many cases of nonspecific itching.

Yellow Jasmine *(Gelsemium sempervirens)*

The rhizome and roots contain a volatile oil, a resin, an alkaloid, and an acid. *Gelsemium* is a depressant to the circulatory, nervous, and respiratory systems. It is used to treat headaches, migraine, early stages of pneumonia, asthma, whopping cough, and other spasmodic conditions. In fluidextract, the dose is usually ½ to 2 minims, and in tincture, 5 to 15 minims. It is toxic in large doses.

Yoga

A method of achieving harmony between the self and the source of spiritual power. It consists of meditation, contemplation, and absorption. Four of the six yogas are: *bhakti yoga,* the seeking of a pathway through devotion and love; *mantra yoga,* primarily linked with the worship of Krishna and principally concerned with the vibrations and radiations of life much associated with musical-minded seekers; *karma yoga,* the seeking of the pathway through service to others. This is service in action and it emphasizes the need to live in the present world and make the best of it; and *inana yoga,* the seeking of the path through the aspiration of the intellect. The 3HO Foundation operates many centers in the United States under the direction of Yogi Bhajan. His center in Tucson, Arizona, developed a program of curing drug addiction which to date has been the most successful method of therapy. The 3HO Drug Program, located at 1050 North Cherry, Tucson, Arizona 85722, in 1978 was accredited as the first and only hospital for emphasizing totally natural therapeutics in the treatment of drug addiction.

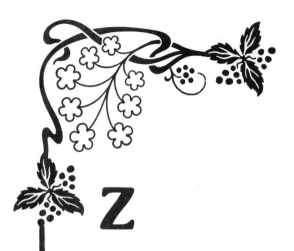

Z

Zinc

Contributing greatly to the efficiency of muscular control by the mind, zinc facilitates coordination of mind and muscle. It aids the metabolism of both proteins and carbohydrates, thus creating energy. It is of value in controlling the storage of both sugars and starches. It aids the respiration of the tissues. Without zinc, there seems to be a decreased efficiency in the manufacture of male hormones, leading to weakness in the reproductive organs. Diabetes has also been related to zinc deficiency, due to its effect upon the storage of sugar. Constipation over long periods often indicates a shortage of zinc. Zinc is found in beans, egg yolk, most legumes, most nuts, peas, the green leaves of vegetables, and above all, in wheat germ. Since zinc is found in most green leaves, it is found in abundance in many herbs.

Zone Therapy (See *Reflexology*)

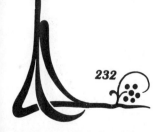

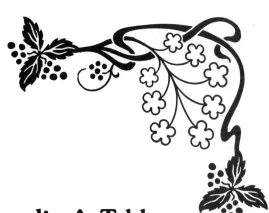

Appendix A: Tables

Appendix A—Tables

Digestion Time of Foods

1¼ hours
parsley

1½ hours
lemon
agar
Irish moss

1¾ hours
avocado
grapes
mango
olive, ripe
raspberry

2 hours
blueberry
sweet cherry
grapefruit
orange
raisin
coconut milk
artichoke, globe
beet greens
garlic
potato
tomato
brown rice

2¼ hours
fig, fresh
pear, fresh
pineapple
strawberry
asparagus
carrot
cauliflower

lettuce: cos,
      loose leaf,
      iceberg

2½ hours
blackberry
date
fig, dried
gooseberry
peach, fresh
almond
dandelion greens
leek
mushroom
okra
lima bean
white rice

2¾ hours
apple, fresh
apricot, fresh
currant
peach, dried
plum
watermelon
chestnut
coconut meat, fresh
pecan
pignolia
beet
dock (sorrel)
summer squash
wheat bran

3 hours
banana
guava

lime
prune, dried
beechnut
filbert
walnut
broccoli
common cabbage
Swiss chard
sweet corn
endive (escarole)
kohlrabi
rhubarb
spinach
winter squash
white bean
lentil
soybean
wheat germ

3¼ hours
cranberry
cantaloupe
casaba melon
honeydew melon
olive oil
pomegranate
cashew nut
coconut meat, dried
celery
cucumber
onion
sweet green pepper
pumpkin

radish
rutabaga
sweet potato
turnip greens
watercress
snap bean
cowpea
pea, fresh
peanut
millet

3½ hours
safflower seed oil
sesame seed oil
celeriac
eggplant
mustard greens
parsnip
pea, dried
soybean oil
rye grain

3¾ hours
persimmon
quince
red cabbage
barley
wheat grain

4 hours
brussels sprouts
horseradish
turnip

Source: Composition and Facts about Foods, Ford Heritage, Mokelumne Hill,
Calif.: Health Research, 1971.

Composition of Blood

Constituent	Average Value* per 100 milligrams of Blood
hemoglobin, male(B)**	15.9 grams
total protein (S)	7.2 grams
albumin (S)	5.2 grams
globulin (S)	2.0 grams
nonprotein nitrogen (B)	29.0 milligrams
urea nitrogen (B)	13.6 milligrams
creatinine (P)	1.0 milligrams
uric acid (S)	4.4 milligrams
glucose (B)	90.0 milligrams
CO_2 capacity (P)	60% by volume
cholesterol, total (S)	210.0 milligrams
calcium (S)	10.0 milligrams
phosphorus (S)	3.6 milligrams
NaCl (P)	595.0 milligrams
bilirubin (S)	0.54 milligrams

*Most of these values were taken from *Biochemistry of Disease,* by Bodansky and Bodansky, 2nd ed. New York: Macmillan, 1952.

**B=whole blood; S=serum; P=plasm.

Dry Measures

Avoirdupois

1 grain	=	0.06 grams		
1 dram	=	27.3 grains	=	1.77 grams
1 ounce	=	16 drams	=	28.35 grams
1 pound	=	16 ounces	=	4.53 grams

Apothecary (Troy)

1 scruple	=	20 grains	=	1.30 grams
1 dram	=	3 scruples	=	3.89 grams
1 ounce	=	8 drams	=	37.10 grams
1 pound	=	12 ounces	=	3.73 grams

Metric

1 centigram	=	10 milligrams	=	0.15 grains
1 decigram	=	10 centigrams	=	1.54 grains
1 gram	=	10 decigrams	=	15.43 grains
1 decagram	=	10 grams	=	0.35 ounces
1 hectogram	=	10 decagrams	=	3.53 ounces
1 kilogram	=	10 hectograms	=	2.20 pounds

Liquid Measures

U.S.

1 teaspoon				5 milliliters
1 tablespoon	=	½ fluidounce	=	15 milliliters
1 ounce	=	2 tablespoons	=	0.03 liters
1 gill	=	4 fluidounces	=	0.12 liters
1 cup	=	8 fluidounces	=	0.24 liters
1 pint	=	2 cups	=	0.48 liters
1 quart	=	2 pints	=	0.96 liters
1 gallon	=	4 quarts	=	3.78 liters

Metric

1 centiliter	=	10 milliliters	=	0.34 fluid ounces
1 deciliter	=	10 centiliters	=	3.38 fluid ounces
1 liter	=	10 deciliters	=	1.06 quarts
1 decaliter	=	10 liters	=	2.64 gallons

Apothecary

1 minim	=	0.06 milliliters	=	approximately one drop from an eyedropper
1 fluidram	=	60 minims	=	3.70 milliliters

Household Measures

Household	Apothecary	Metric
less than a teaspoon	= a few grains	
teaspoon	= 1 dram	= 4 cubic centimeters
dessert spoon	= 2 drams	= 8 cubic centimeters
tablespoon	= 4 drams	= 15 cubic centimeters
teacup	= 6 ounces	= 200 cubic centimeters
tumbler	= 8 ounces	= 250 cubic centimeters
fruit jar	= ½ pint, 1 pint	= 250, 500 cubic centimeters
	1 quart, ½ gallon	= 1000, 2000 cubic centimeters

Approximate Equivalents
Between Apothecary and Metric Systems

Apothecary		Metric
1/60th grain	=	1 milligram
1 grain	=	60 milligrams
15 grains	=	1 gram
15 or 16 minims	=	1 gram
1 dram	=	4 grams
1 ounce	=	30 grams
1 pint	=	475–500 grams

Appendix B:
Composition of Foods

Appendix B—Composition of Foods

Fruit	Water %	Energy Calories	Carbohydrates Total Gms	Fiber Gms	Fat Gms	Total Fatty Acids Sat'd Gms	Unsaturated Oleic Gms	Linol Gms	Protein Gms	Ash Gms	Organic Acids Citric %	Malic %	Oxalic %	pH	Metab React Alkal (Acid)	Digest Time Hrs
Acerola cherry	92.3	28	6.8	.4	.3	—	—	—	.4	.2	—	—	—	—	—	—
Acerola juice	94.3	23	4.8	.3	.3	—	—	—	.4	.2	—	—	—	—	—	—
Apple, not pared	84.8	56	14.1	1.0	.6	—	—	—	.2	.3	trace	.71	0	3.55	2.2	2¾
Apple pared	85.3	53	13.9	.6	.3	—	—	—	.2	.3	—	—	—	—	—	—
Apple dried	24.0	275	71.8	3.1	1.6	—	—	—	1.0	1.6	—	—	—	—	—	—
Apple juice	87.8	47	11.9	.1	trace	—	—	—	.1	.2	—	—	—	—	—	—
Apricot, fresh	85.3	51	12.8	.6	.2	—	—	—	1.0	.7	—	—	.0140	4.40	6.6	2¾
Apricot, dried	25.0	260	66.5	3.0	.5	—	—	—	5.0	3.0	0.35	.81	0	—	36.6	—
Avocado, Calif.	73.6	171	6.0	1.5	17.0	3	8	2	2.2	1.2	0	0	0	6.42	10.7	1¾
Avocado, Fla.	78.0	128	8.8	1.5	11.0	2	5	1	1.3	.9	0	0	0	6.42	10.7	1¾
Banana, common	75.7	85	22.2	.5	.2	—	—	—	1.1	.8	.23	.37	.0064	5.12	6.0	3
Banana, red	74.4	90	23.4	.4	.2	—	—	—	1.2	.8	—	—	—	4.65	—	—
Banana, dehydrated	3.0	340	88.6	2.0	.8	—	—	—	4.4	3.2	—	—	—	—	—	—
Blackberry	84.5	58	12.9	4.1	.9	—	—	—	1.2	.5	trace	.16	.0180	4.30	7.7	2½
Blueberry	83.2	62	15.3	1.5	.5	—	—	—	.7	.3	1.56	.10	.0150	3.21	(1.4)	2
Breadfruit	70.8	103	26.2	1.2	.3	—	—	—	1.7	1.0	—	—	—	—	—	—
Carambola	90.4	35	8.0	.9	.5	—	—	—	.7	.4	—	—	—	—	—	—
Carissa (natalplum)	80.8	70	16.0	.9	1.3	—	—	—	.5	.4	—	—	—	—	—	—
Cherimoya	73.5	94	24.0	2.2	.4	—	—	—	1.3	.8	—	—	—	—	—	—
Cherry, sour red	83.7	58	14.3	.2	.3	—	—	—	1.2	.5	.01	—	.0011	3.17	4.1	—
Cherry, sweet	80.4	70	17.4	.4	.3	—	—	—	1.3	.6	0	.93	0	4.16	7.3	2
Crabapple	81.1	68	17.8	.6	.3	—	—	—	.4	.4	—	—	—	—	—	—
Cranberry	87.9	46	10.8	1.4	.7	—	—	—	.4	.2	1.46	.36	—	3.20	—	3¾
Currant, black	84.2	54	13.1	2.4	.1	—	—	—	1.7	.9	2.30	.05	—	6.00	—	2¾
Currant, red-white	85.7	50	12.1	3.4	.2	—	—	—	1.4	.6	—	—	.0190	4.80	—	2¾
Custardapple	71.5	101	25.2	3.4	.6	—	—	—	1.7	1.0	—	—	—	—	—	—

Fruit	Water %	Energy Calories	Carbohydrates Total Gms	Fiber Gms	Fat Gms	Total Fatty Acids Sat'd Gms	Unsaturated Oleic Gms	Linol Gms	Protein Gms	Ash Gms	Organic Acids Citric %	Malic %	Oxalic %	pH	Metab React Alkal (Acid)	Digest Time Hrs
Date	22.5	274	72.9	2.3	.5	—	—	—	2.2	1.9	—	—	—	4.77	9.6	2½
Elderberry	79.8	72	16.4	7.0	.5	—	—	—	2.6	.7	—	—	—	—	—	—
Fig, fresh	77.5	80	20.3	1.2	.3	—	—	—	1.2	.7	.34	trace	—	5.12	—	2¼
Fig, dried	23.0	274	69.1	5.6	1.3	—	—	—	4.3	2.3	—	—	—	—	43.7	2½
Gooseberry	88.9	39	9.7	1.9	.2	—	—	—	.8	.4	trace	1.29	.0880	—	5.5	2½
Granadilla (passion fruit)	75.1	90	21.2	—	.7	—	—	—	2.2	.8	—	—	—	—	8.5	—
Grapefruit, pulp	88.4	41	10.6	.2	.1	—	—	—	.5	.4	1.40	.08	.0150	3.45	6.4	2
Grapefruit, juice	90.0	39	9.2	trace	.1	—	—	—	.5	.4	—	—	—	—	—	—
Grapes, American type (slip skin) Concord, Delaware, etc.	81.6	69	15.7	.6	1.3	—	—	—	1.3	.4	—	.65	.0250	2.89	2.7	1¾
Grapes, European type (adherent skin) Malaga, Muscat, Thompson seedless, Emperor, etc.	81.4	67	17.3	.5	.3	—	—	—	.6	.4	—	—	.0130	3.59	2.7	1¾
Groundcherry	85.4	53	11.2	2.8	.7	—	—	—	1.9	.8	—	—	—	—	—	—
Guava, common	83.0	62	15.0	5.6	.6	—	—	—	.8	.6	—	—	—	—	7.7	3
Guava, strawberry	81.8	65	15.8	6.4	.6	—	—	—	1.0	.8	—	—	—	—	—	—
Haw, scarlet	75.8	87	20.8	2.1	.7	—	—	—	2.0	.8	—	—	—	—	—	—
Jackfruit	72.0	98	25.4	1.0	.3	—	—	—	1.3	1.0	—	—	—	—	—	—
Jujube, fresh	70.2	105	27.6	1.4	.2	—	—	—	1.2	.8	—	—	—	—	—	—
Jujube, dried	19.7	287	73.6	3.0	1.1	—	—	—	3.7	1.9	—	—	—	—	—	—
Kumquat	81.3	65	17.1	3.7	.1	—	—	—	.9	.6	—	—	—	3.85	—	—
Lemon, peeled	90.1	27	8.2	.4	.3	—	—	—	1.1	.3	3.84	trace	—	—	7.7	1½
Lemon, with peel	87.4	20	10.7	—	.3	—	—	—	1.2	.4	—	.29	—	—	8.5	—
Lemon, juice	91.0	25	8.0	trace	.2	—	—	—	.5	.3	6.08	—	0	2.04	4.0	—

Fruit	Water %	Energy Calories	Carbohydrates Total Gms	Carbohydrates Fiber Gms	Fat Gms	Total Fatty Acids Sat'd Gms	Unsaturated Oleic Gms	Unsaturated Linol Gms	Protein Gms	Ash Gms	Organic Acids Citric %	Organic Acids Malic %	Organic Acids Oxalic %	pH	Metab React Alkal (Acid)	Digest Time Hrs
Lime	89.3	28	9.5	.5	.2	—	—	—	.7	.3	—	—	.1100	—	—	3
Lime, juice	90.3	26	9.0	trace	.1	—	—	—	.3	.3	—	—	0	2.10	—	—
Loganberry	83.0	62	14.9	3.0	.6	—	—	—	1.0	.5	2.02	.08	—	—	7.4	—
Longan, fresh	82.4	61	15.8	.4	.1	—	—	—	1.0	.7	—	—	—	—	—	—
Longan, dried	17.6	286	74.0	2.0	.4	—	—	—	4.9	3.1	—	—	—	—	—	—
Loquat	86.5	48	12.4	.5	.2	—	—	—	.4	.5	—	—	—	—	—	—
Lychee, fresh	81.9	64	16.4	.3	.3	—	—	—	.9	.5	—	—	—	—	—	—
Lychee, dried	22.3	277	70.7	1.4	1.2	—	—	—	3.8	2.0	—	—	—	—	—	—
Mamey	86.2	51	12.5	1.0	.5	—	—	—	.5	.3	—	—	—	—	5.0	—
Mango	81.7	66	16.8	.9	.4	—	—	—	.7	.4	—	—	0	4.17	5.0	1¾
Muskmelons:																
Cantaloupe	91.2	30	7.5	.3	.1	—	—	—	.7	.5	0	—	0	6.52	7.5	3¼
Casaba	91.5	27	6.5	.5	trace	—	—	—	1.2	.8	—	—	0	5.73	—	3¼
Honeydew	90.6	33	7.7	.6	.3	—	—	—	.8	.6	—	—	0	6.38	—	3¼
Nectarine	81.8	64	17.1	.4	trace	—	—	—	.6	.5	—	—	0	3.99	6.2	—
Olive, pickled:																
Green	78.2	116	1.3	1.3	12.7	2	10	1	1.4	6.4	—	—	—	—	(3.8)	—
Ripe, Ascolano	80.0	129	2.6	1.4	13.8	2	15	1	1.1	2.5	—	—	—	6.00	—	1¾
Ripe, Mission	73.0	184	3.2	1.5	20.1	1	7	1	1.2	2.5	—	—	—	6.00	—	1¾
Ripe, Sevillano	84.4	93	2.7	1.2	9.5	—	—	—	1.1	2.3	—	—	—	6.00	—	1¾
Olive oil	0	884	0	0	100.0	11	76	7	—	—	—	—	—	—	—	3¼
Orange, peeled	86.0	49	12.2	.5	.2	—	—	—	1.0	.6	.95	.09	.0240	3.90	7.1	2
Orange, with peel	82.3	40	15.5	—	.3	—	—	—	1.3	.6	—	—	.0780	—	—	—
Orange, peel only	72.5	—	25.0	—	.2	—	—	—	1.5	.8	—	—	—	—	—	—
Orange juice	88.3	45	10.4	.1	.2	—	—	—	.7	.4	—	—	—	—	0.1	—
Papaw	76.6	85	16.8	—	.9	—	—	—	5.2	.5	—	—	—	3.76	4.5	—
Papaya	88.7	39	10.0	.9	.1	—	—	—	.6	.6	—	—	—	5.49	—	—

Fruit	Water %	Energy Calories	Carbohydrates Total Gms	Carbohydrates Fiber Gms	Fat Gms	Total Fatty Acids: Total Sat'd Gms	Total Fatty Acids: Unsaturated Oleic Gms	Total Fatty Acids: Unsaturated Linol Gms	Protein Gms	Ash Gms	Organic Acids: Citric %	Organic Acids: Malic %	Organic Acids: Oxalic %	pH	Metab React Alkal (Acid)	Digest Time Hrs
Peach, fresh	89.1	38	9.7	.6	.1	—	—	—	.6	.5	.37	.37	.0025	3.57	8.2	2½
Peach, dried	25.0	262	68.3	3.1	.7	—	—	—	3.1	2.9	—	—	—	—	12.1	2¾
Pear, fresh	83.2	61	15.3	1.4	.4	—	—	—	.7	.4	.24	.12	.0030	3.92	3.4	2¼
Pear, dried	26.0	268	67.3	6.2	1.8	—	—	—	3.1	1.8	—	—	—	—	—	—
Persimmon, kaki	78.6	77	19.7	1.6	.4	—	—	—	.7	.6	—	.09	—	5.53	—	3¾
Persimmon, native	64.4	127	33.5	1.5	.4	—	—	—	.8	.9	—	—	—	5.53	—	3¾
Pineapple	85.3	52	13.7	.4	.2	—	—	—	.4	.4	.80	.12	—	3.44	5.8	2¼
Pitanga (surinam cherry)	85.8	51	12.5	.6	.4	—	—	—	.8	.5	—	—	—	—	—	—
Plantain	66.4	119	31.2	.4	.4	—	—	—	1.1	.9	—	—	—	—	—	—
Plum, Damson	81.1	66	17.8	.4	trace	—	—	—	.5	.6	0	2.48	.0100	3.00	8.2	2¾
Plum, Japanese	86.6	48	12.3	.6	.2	—	—	—	.5	.4	—	—	—	—	—	2¾
Plum, prune type	78.7	75	19.7	.4	.2	—	—	—	.8	.6	—	—	—	3.05	—	2¾
Pomegranate pulp	82.3	63	16.4	.2	.3	—	—	—	.5	.5	4.52	0	—	3.00	3.5	3¼
Pricklypear	88.0	42	10.9	1.6	.1	—	—	—	.5	.5	—	—	—	—	6.7	—
Prune, dried	28.0	255	67.4	1.6	.6	—	—	—	2.1	1.9	0	1.44	.0058	—	20.3	3
Prune, dehydrated	2.8	344	91.3	2.2	.5	—	—	—	3.3	2.4	—	—	—	—	—	—
Quince	83.8	57	15.3	1.7	.1	—	—	—	.4	.4	0	1.13	—	—	4.9	3¾
Raisin	18.0	289	77.4	.9	.2	—	—	—	2.5	1.9	—	—	—	3.95	25.3	2
Raspberry, black	80.8	73	15.7	5.1	1.4	—	—	—	1.5	.6	1.06	—	.0530	3.73	5.7	1¾
Raspberry, red	84.2	57	13.6	3.0	.5	—	—	—	1.2	.5	1.30	.04	.0150	3.73	5.7	1¾
Roseapple	84.5	56	14.2	1.1	.3	—	—	—	.6	.4	—	—	—	—	—	—
Sapodilla	76.1	89	21.8	1.4	1.1	—	—	—	.5	.5	—	—	—	—	4.8	—
Sapote	64.9	125	31.6	1.9	.6	—	—	—	1.8	1.1	—	—	—	—	—	—
Soursop	81.7	65	16.3	1.1	.3	—	—	—	1.0	.7	—	—	—	—	—	—
Strawberry	89.9	37	8.4	1.3	.5	—	—	—	.7	.5	1.00	.13	.0190	3.43	2.6	2¼

	Water %	Energy Calories	Carbohydrates Total Gms	Fiber Gms	Fat Gms	Total Sat'd Gms	Unsaturated Oleic Gms	Linol Gms	Protein Gms	Ash Gms	Citric %	Malic %	Oxalic %	pH	Metab React Alkal (Acid)	Digest Time Hrs
Fruit																
Sugarapple (sweetsop)	73.3	94	23.7	1.7	.3	—	—	—	1.8	.9	—	—	—	—	—	—
Tamarind	31.4	239	62.5	5.1	.6	—	—	—	2.8	2.7	trace	.50	—	—	—	—
Tangelo juice	89.4	41	9.7	trace	.1	—	—	—	.5	.3	—	—	—	—	—	—
Tangerine	87.0	46	11.6	.5	.2	—	—	—	.8	.4	—	—	—	4.10	5.7	—
Tangerine juice	88.9	43	10.1	.1	.2	—	—	—	.5	.3	—	—	—	—	—	—
Towelgourd	94.5	18	4.1	.5	.2	—	—	—	.8	.4	—	—	0	—	—	—
Watermelon	92.6	26	6.4	.3	.2	—	—	—	.5	.3	—	.20	0	5.33	2.2	2¾
Waxgourd	96.1	13	3.0	.5	.2	—	—	—	.4	.3	—	—	—	—	—	—
Seed																
Pumpkin & Squash	4.4	553	15.0	1.9	46.7	8	17	20	29.0	4.9	—	—	—	—	—	—
Safflower	5.0	615	12.4	—	59.5	5	9	43	19.1	4.0	—	—	—	—	—	—
Safflower, oil	0	884	0	0	100.0	8	15	72	0	0	—	—	—	—	—	3½
Sesame, whole	5.4	563	21.6	6.3	49.1	7	19	21	18.6	5.3	—	—	—	—	—	—
Sesame, hulled	5.5	582	17.6	2.4	53.4	7	20	22	18.2	5.3	—	—	—	—	—	—
Sesame, oil	0	884	0	0	100.0	14	38	42	0	0	—	—	—	—	—	3½
Sunflower	4.8	560	19.9	3.8	47.3	6	9	30	24.0	4.0	—	—	—	—	—	—
Sunflower, oil	0	884	0	0	100.0	13	21	66	0	0	—	—	—	—	—	3½

Nut	Water %	Energy Calories	Carbohydrates Total Gms	Carbohydrates Fiber Gms	Fat Gms	Total Sat'd Gms	Unsaturated Oleic Gms	Unsaturated Linol Gms	Protein Gms	Ash Gms	Citric %	Malic %	Oxalic %	pH	Metab React Alkal (Acid)	Digest Time Hrs
Almond	4.7	598	19.5	2.6	54.2	4	36	11	18.6	3.0	—	—	.4100	—	13.5	2½
Beechnut	6.6	568	20.3	3.7	50.0	4	27	16	19.4	3.7	—	—	—	—	—	3
Brazilnut	4.6	654	10.9	3.1	66.9	13	32	17	14.3	3.3	—	—	—	—	(3.2)	—
Butternut	3.8	629	8.4	—	61.2	8	32	3	23.7	2.9	—	—	—	—	—	—
Cashew	5.2	561	29.3	1.4	45.7	8	32	3	17.2	2.6	—	—	.3200	—	—	3¼
Chestnut, fresh	52.5	194	42.1	1.1	1.5	—	—	—	2.9	1.0	—	—	—	—	9.1	2¾
Chestnut, dried	8.4	377	78.6	2.5	4.1	—	—	—	6.7	2.2	—	—	—	—	—	—
Coconut cream	54.1	334	8.3	—	32.2	28	2	trace	4.4	1.0	—	—	—	—	—	2¾
Coconut, meat	50.9	346	9.4	4.0	35.3	30	2	trace	3.5	.9	—	—	—	6.10	6.0	3¼
Coconut, meat, dry	3.5	662	23.0	3.9	64.9	56	5	trace	7.2	1.4	—	—	—	—	8.5	2
Coconut, milk	65.7	252	5.2	—	24.9	22	2	trace	3.2	1.0	—	—	—	—	7.5	—
Coconut, water	94.2	22	4.7	trace	.2	—	—	—	.3	.6	—	—	—	5.04	—	—
Filbert	5.8	634	16.7	3.0	62.4	3	34	10	12.6	2.5	—	—	—	—	(2.1)	3
Hickory	3.3	673	12.8	1.9	68.7	6	47	12	13.2	2.0	—	—	—	—	—	—
Macadamia	3.0	691	15.9	2.5	71.6	—	—	—	7.8	1.7	—	—	—	—	—	2¾
Pecan	3.4	687	14.6	2.3	71.2	5	45	14	9.2	1.6	—	—	—	—	—	2¾
Pignolia	5.6	552	11.6	.9	47.4	—	—	—	31.1	4.3	—	—	—	—	—	—
Pilinut	6.3	669	8.4	2.7	71.1	—	—	—	11.4	2.8	—	—	—	—	—	—
Pinon	3.1	635	20.5	1.1	60.5	—	—	—	13.0	2.9	—	—	—	—	—	—
Pistachio	5.3	594	19.0	1.9	53.7	5	35	10	19.3	2.7	—	—	—	—	—	—
Walnut, black	3.1	628	14.8	1.7	59.3	4	21	28	20.5	2.3	—	—	—	—	—	3
Walnut, English	3.5	651	15.8	2.1	64.0	4	10	40	14.8	1.9	—	—	—	5.42	(8.5)	3
Waterchestnut, Chinese	78.3	79	19.0	.8	.2	—	—	—	1.4	1.1	—	—	—	—	(0.2)	—

Vegetable	Water %	Energy Calories	Carbohydrates Total Gms	Fiber Gms	Fat Gms	Total Sat'd Gms	Unsaturated Oleic Gms	Linol Gms	Protein Gms	Ash Gms	Citric %	Malic %	Oxalic %	pH	Metab React Alkal (Acid)	Digest Time Hrs
Artichoke, globe	85.5	9-47	10.6	2.4	.2	—	—	—	2.9	.8	.10	.17	—	—	(4.3)	2
Asparagus	91.7	26	5.0	.7	.2	—	—	—	2.5	.6	.11	.10	.0052	—	(0.1)	2¼
Bamboo shoots	91.0	27	5.2	.7	.3	—	—	—	2.6	.9	—	—	—	—	7.7	—
Beet, common red	87.3	43	9.9	.8	.1	—	—	—	1.6	1.1	.11	0	.1380	—	11.1	2¾
Beet, greens	90.9	24	4.6	1.3	.3	—	—	—	2.2	2.0	—	—	.9160	—	—	2
Broccoli	89.1	32	5.9	1.5	.3	—	—	—	3.6	1.1	.21	.12	.0054	—	4.2	3
Brussels sprouts	85.2	45	8.3	1.6	.4	—	—	—	4.9	1.2	.24	.20	.0059	—	4.3	4
Cabbage, Chinese	95.0	14	3.0	.6	.1	—	—	—	1.2	.7	—	—	.0073	6.16	—	—
Cabbage, common	92.4	24	5.4	.8	.2	—	—	—	1.3	.7	.14	.10	.0077	6.03	6.2	3
Cabbage, red	90.2	31	6.9	1.0	.2	—	—	—	2.0	.7	—	—	—	5.78	3.9	3¾
Cabbage, savoy	92.0	24	4.6	.8	.2	—	—	—	2.4	.8	—	—	—	—	2.7	—
Cabbage, spoon	94.3	16	2.9	.6	.2	—	—	—	1.6	1.0	—	—	—	—	—	—
Carrot	88.2	42	9.7	1.0	.2	—	—	—	1.1	.8	.09	.24	.0330	5.97	10.2	2¼
Cauliflower	91.0	27	5.2	1.0	.2	—	—	—	2.7	.9	.21	.39	0	—	3.2	2¼
Celeriac	88.4	40	8.5	1.3	.3	—	—	—	1.8	1.0	—	—	—	—	—	3½
Celery	94.1	17	3.9	.6	.1	—	—	—	.9	1.0	.01	.17	.0560	5.89	8.1	3¼
Chard, Swiss	91.1	25	4.6	.8	.3	—	—	—	2.4	1.6	—	—	.6450	—	20.4	3
Chayote	91.8	28	7.1	.7	.1	—	—	—	.6	.4	—	—	—	—	—	—
Chervil	80.7	57	11.5	—	.9	—	—	—	3.4	3.5	—	—	—	—	—	—
Chicory	95.1	15	3.2	—	.1	—	—	—	1.0	.6	—	—	—	5.97	3.2	—
Chicory, greens	92.8	20	3.8	.8	.3	—	—	—	1.8	1.3	—	—	—	—	—	—
Chive	91.3	28	5.8	1.1	.3	—	—	—	1.8	.8	—	—	—	5.81	10.4	—
Collards, leaves	85.3	45	7.5	1.2	.8	—	—	—	4.8	1.6	—	—	.0091	—	—	—
Collards, leaves and stems	86.9	40	7.2	.9	.7	—	—	—	3.6	1.6	—	—	—	—	—	—
Corn, sweet	72.7	96	22.1	.7	1.0	—	—	—	3.5	.7	0	0	.0033	—	1.8	3
Corn, oil	0	884	0	0	100.0	10	28	53	0	0	—	—	—	—	—	3½

Vegetable	Water %	Energy Calories	Carbohydrates Total Gms	Carbohydrates Fiber Gms	Fat Gms	Total Fatty Acids Total Sat'd Gms	Total Fatty Acids Unsaturated Oleic Gms	Total Fatty Acids Linol Gms	Protein Gms	Ash Gms	Organic Acids Citric %	Organic Acids Malic %	Organic Acids Oxalic %	pH	Metab React Alkal (Acid)	Digest Time Hrs
Cress	89.4	32	5.5	1.1	.7	—	—	—	2.6	1.8	—	—	.0053	—	(2.3)	—
Cucumber w/skin	95.1	15	3.4	.6	.1	—	—	—	.9	.5	.01	.24	0	5.48	14.2	3¼
Dandelion greens	85.6	45	9.2	1.6	.7	—	—	—	2.7	1.8	—	—	.0246	—	17.5	2½
Dock (sorrel)	90.9	28	5.6	.8	.3	—	—	—	2.1	1.1	—	—	—	3.12	—	2¾
Eggplant	92.4	25	5.6	.9	.2	—	—	—	1.2	.6	0	.17	.0069	—	4.5	3½
Endive (escarole)	93.1	20	4.1	.9	.1	—	—	—	1.7	1.0	—	—	.0273	5.90	9.9	3
Fennel	90.0	28	5.1	.5	.4	—	—	—	2.8	1.7	—	—	—	5.91	—	—
Garlic	61.3	137	30.8	1.5	.2	—	—	—	6.2	1.5	—	—	—	—	—	2
Horseradish, raw	74.6	87	19.7	2.4	.3	—	—	—	3.2	2.2	—	—	—	5.35	4.2	4
Horseradish, prepared	87.1	38	9.6	.9	.2	—	—	—	1.3	1.8	—	—	—	3.56	—	—
Jerusalem artichoke	79.8	7-75	16.7	.8	.1	—	—	—	2.3	1.1	—	—	—	—	(10.3)	—
Kale, leaves	82.7	53	9.0	—	.8	—	—	—	6.0	1.5	.35	.05	.0110	—	10.5	—
Kale Leaf & stem	87.5	38	6.0	1.3	.8	—	—	—	4.2	1.5	—	—	.0130	—	—	—
Kohlrabi	90.3	29	6.6	1.0	.1	—	—	—	2.0	1.0	—	—	—	—	6.0	3
Leek	85.4	52	11.2	1.3	.3	—	—	—	2.2	.9	—	—	—	5.77	7.3	2½
Lettuce:																
Boston, Bibb	95.1	14	2.5	.5	.2	—	—	—	1.2	1.0	—	—	—	5.99	—	—
Cos, Looseleaf	94.0	18	3.5	.7	.3	—	—	—	1.3	.9	—	—	—	5.95	7.0	2¼
Iceberg, N.Y.	95.5	13	2.9	.5	.1	—	—	—	.9	.6	.02	.17	.0071	5.93	7.7	2¼
Mushroom	90.4	28	4.4	.8	.3	—	—	—	2.7	.9	0	.14	—	—	4.9	2½
Mustard greens	89.5	31	5.6	1.1	.5	—	—	—	3.0	1.4	—	—	.0077	—	—	3½
Mustard spinach	92.2	22	3.9	1.0	.3	—	—	—	2.2	1.4	—	—	—	—	—	—
N.Z. spinach	92.6	19	3.1	.7	.3	—	—	—	2.2	1.8	—	—	.8900	—	—	—
Okra	88.9	36	7.6	1.0	.3	—	—	—	2.4	.8	.02	.12	.0480	—	4.5	2½

Vegetable	Water %	Energy Calories	Carbohydrates Total Gms	Fiber Gms	Fat Gms	Total Fatty Acids Total Sat'd Gms	Unsaturated Oleic Gms	Linol Gms	Protein Gms	Ash Gms	Citric %	Malic %	Oxalic %	pH	Metab React Alkal (Acid)	Digest Time Hrs
Onion, green	89.4	36	8.2	1.2	.2	—	—	—	1.5	.7	—	—	.0230	—	8.4	—
Onion, mature dry	89.1	38	8.7	.6	.1	—	—	—	1.5	.6	.02	.17	—	5.49	—	3¼
Onion, Welsh	90.5	34	6.5	1.0	.4	—	—	—	1.9	.7	—	—	—	—	—	1¼
Parsley	85.1	44	8.5	1.5	.6	—	—	—	3.6	2.2	—	—	.1900	5.85	—	3½
Parsnip	79.1	76	17.5	2.0	.5	—	—	—	1.7	1.2	.13	.35	.0100	—	8.6	
Pepper:																
Hot green	88.8	37	9.1	1.8	.2	—	—	—	1.3	.6	—	—	—	—	—	—
Hot red raw	74.3	93	18.1	9.0	2.3	—	—	—	3.7	1.6	—	—	—	—	—	—
Hot red dry	12.6	321	59.8	26.2	9.1	—	—	—	12.9	7.4	—	—	—	—	—	3¼
Sweet green	93.4	22	4.8	1.4	.2	—	—	—	1.2	.4	—	—	.0160	5.49	—	—
Sweet red	90.7	31	7.1	1.7	.3	—	—	—	1.4	.5	—	—	—	—	7.2	2
Potato w/skin	79.8	76	17.1	.5	.1	—	—	—	2.1	.9	.51	0	.0057	—	3.2	3¼
Pumpkin	91.6	26	6.5	1.1	.1	—	—	—	1.0	.8	0	.15	—	—	—	—
Purslane leaves	92.5	21	3.8	.9	.4	—	—	—	1.7	1.6	—	—	.9100	—	4.8	3¼
Radish, common	94.5	17	3.6	.7	.1	—	—	—	1.0	.8	—	—	0	5.72	—	—
Radish, oriental	94.1	19	4.2	.7	.1	—	—	—	.9	.7	—	—	—	—	10.2	3
Rhubarb	94.8	16	3.7	.7	.1	—	—	—	.6	.8	.41	1.77	.5000	—	8.5	3¼
Rutabaga	87.0	46	11.0	1.1	.1	—	—	—	1.1	.8	—	—	—	—	—	1½
Salsify	77.6	13-82	18.0	1.8	.6	—	—	—	2.9	.9	—	—	—	—	—	—
Seaweed, agar	16.3	—	—	.7	.3	—	—	—	—	3.7	—	—	—	—	—	—
Seaweed, dulse	16.6	—	44.2	1.2	3.2	—	—	—	25.3	22.4	—	—	—	—	—	1½
Seaweed, irishmos	19.2	—	—	2.1	1.8	—	—	—	—	17.6	—	—	—	—	—	—
Seaweed, kelp	21.7	—	40.2	6.8	1.1	—	—	—	7.5	22.8	—	—	—	—	—	—
Seaweed, laver	17.0	—	—	3.5	.6	—	—	—	—	11.0	—	—	—	—	—	—
Shallot	79.8	72	16.8	.7	.1	—	—	—	2.5	.8	.08	.09	.8920	—	15.8	—
Spinach	90.7	26	4.3	.6	.3	—	—	—	3.2	1.5	—	—	—	—	—	3

Vegetable	Water %	Energy Calories	Carbohydrates Total Gms	Carbohydrates Fiber Gms	Fat Gms	Total Fatty Acids Total Sat'd Gms	Unsaturated Oleic Gms	Unsaturated Linol Gms	Protein Gms	Ash Gms	Organic Acids Citric %	Malic %	Oxalic %	pH	Metab React Alkal (Acid)	Digest Time Hrs
Squash:																
Summer (yellow, scallop and zucchini)	94.0	19	4.2	.6	.1	—	—	—	1.1	.6	.04	.32	0	—	—	2¾
Winter (Acorn, butternut and hubbard)	85.1	50	12.4	1.4	.3	—	—	—	1.4	.8	—	—	—	—	2.8	3
Swamp cabbage	89.7	29	5.4	1.1	.3	—	—	—	3.0	1.6	—	—	—	—	—	—
Sweet potato	70.6	114	26.3	.7	.4	—	—	—	1.7	1.0	.07	0	.0560	—	6.7	3¼
Taro:																
Corms & tubers	73.0	98	23.7	.8	.2	—	—	—	1.9	1.2	—	—	—	—	15.0	—
Leaves & stems	87.2	40	7.4	1.4	.8	—	—	—	3.0	1.6	—	—	—	—	—	—
Tomato, green	93.0	24	5.1	.5	.2	—	—	—	1.2	.5	—	—	—	—	—	—
Tomato, red ripe	93.5	22	4.7	.5	.2	—	—	—	1.1	.5	.38	.12	.0075	4.24	8.3	2
Turnip	91.5	30	6.6	.9	.2	—	—	—	1.0	.7	0	.23	.0018	—	6.5	4
Turnip, greens	90.3	28	5.0	.8	.3	—	—	—	3.0	1.4	—	—	—	—	—	3¼
Vinespinach (basella)	93.1	19	3.4	.7	.3	—	—	—	1.8	1.4	—	—	.0146	—	—	—
Watercress	93.3	19	3.0	.7	.3	—	—	—	2.2	1.2	—	—	—	5.97	8.1	3¼
Yam, tuber	73.5	101	23.2	.9	.2	—	—	—	2.1	1.0	—	—	—	—	—	—
Yambean, tuber	85.1	55	12.8	.7	.2	—	—	—	1.4	.5	—	—	—	—	—	—

Fruit	Cal-cium Mgs	Potas-sium Mgs	Sod-ium Mgs	Magne-sium Mgs	Iron Mgs	Phos-phorus Mgs	Chlo-rine Mgs	Sul-fur Mgs	Sili-con Mgs	Iodine Mgs	Bro-mine Mgs	Vita-min A I.U.	Thia-mine (B-1) Mgs	Ribo-flavin (B-2) Mgs	Nia-cin Mgs	Ascor Acid (C) Mgs
Acerola cherry	12	83	8	—	.2	11	—	—	—	—	—	—	.02	.06	.4	1300
Acerola juice	10	—	3	—	.5	9	—	—	—	—	—	—	.02	.06	.4	1600
Apple, not pared	7	110	1	8	.3	10	—	201	142	.009	.15	90	.03	.02	.1	7
Apple, pared	6	110	1	5	.3	10	—	—	—	—	—	40	.03	.02	.1	4
Apple, dried	31	569	5	22	1.6	52	—	—	—	—	—	—	.06	.12	.5	10
Apple, juice	6	101	1	4	.6	9	—	—	—	—	—	—	.01	.02	.1	1
Apricot, fresh	17	281	1	12	.5	23	20	92	280	—	—	2700	.03	.04	.6	10
Apricot, dried	67	979	26	62	5.5	108	—	164	—	—	—	10900	.01	.16	3.3	12
Avocado, Calif.	10	604	4	45	.6	42	645	505	22	—	—	290	.11	.20	1.6	14
Avocado, Florida	10	604	4	45	.6	42	654	505	22	—	—	290	.11	.20	1.6	14
Banana, common	8	370	1	33	.7	26	270	120	80	.012	.54	190	.05	.06	.7	10
Banana, red	10	370	1	33	.8	18	—	—	—	—	—	400	.05	.04	.6	10
Banana, dehydrated	32	1477	4	132	2.8	104	—	—	—	—	—	760	.18	.24	2.8	7
Blackberry	32	170	1	30	.9	19	180	90	—	.020	—	200	.03	.04	.4	21
Blueberry	15	81	1	6	1.0	13	—	144	42	—	—	100	.03	.06	.5	14
Breadfruit	33	439	15	—	1.2	32	150	375	—	—	—	40	.11	.03	.9	29
Carambola	4	192	2	—	1.5	17	—	—	—	—	—	1200	.04	.02	.3	35
Carissa (natalplum)	—	—	—	—	—	—	—	—	—	—	—	40	.04	.06	.2	38
Cherimoya	23	—	—	—	.5	40	274	167	—	—	—	10	.10	.11	1.3	9
Cherry, sour red	22	191	2	14	.4	19	48	176	311	—	—	1000	.05	.06	.4	10
Cherry, sweet	22	191	2	—	.4	19	48	176	311	.003	trace	110	.05	.06	.4	10
Crabapple	6	110	1	—	.3	13	—	—	—	—	—	40	.03	.02	.1	8
Cranberry	14	82	2	8	.5	10	3	—	—	.005	—	40	.03	.02	.1	11
Currant, black	60	372	3	15	1.1	40	8	1420	—	—	.09	230	.05	.05	.3	200
Currant, red-white	32	257	2	15	1.0	23	33	473	—	—	.12	120	.04	.05	.1	41
Custardapple	27	—	—	—	.8	20	—	595	—	—	—	trace	.08	.10	.5	22

Appendix B: Composition of Foods

Fruit	Calcium Mgs	Potassium Mgs	Sodium Mgs	Magnesium Mgs	Iron Mgs	Phosphorus Mgs	Chlorine Mgs	Sulfur Mgs	Silicon Mgs	Iodine Mgs	Bromine Mgs	Vitamin A I.U.	Thiamine (B-1) Mgs	Riboflavin (B-2) Mgs	Niacin Mgs	Ascorbic Acid (C) Mgs
Date	59	648	1	58	3.0	63	390	120	—	.001	—	50	.09	.10	2.2	0
Elderberry	38	300	—	—	1.6	28	—	—	—	—	—	600	.07	.06	.5	36
Fig, fresh	35	194	2	20	.6	22	—	—	—	.004	.18	80	.06	.05	.4	2
Fig, dried	126	640	34	71	3.0	77	100	270	240	—	—	80	.10	.10	.7	0
Gooseberry	18	155	1	9	.5	15	22	171	75	—	—	290	—	—	—	33
Granadilla (passion fruit)	13	348	28	29	1.6	64	—	—	—	—	—	700	trace	.13	1.5	30
Grapefruit, pulp	16	135	1	12	.4	16	40	100	—	.001	.90	80	.04	.02	.2	38
Grapefruit, juice	9	162	1	12	.2	15	—	—	—	—	—	80	.04	.02	.2	38
Grapes, American type (slip skin) Concord, Delaware, etc.	16	158	3	13	.4	12	35	150	60	—	—	100	.05	.03	.3	4
Grapes, European type (adherent skin) Malaga, Muscat, Thompson seedless, Emperor, etc.	12	173	3	6	.4	20	35	150	60	—	.64	100	.05	.03	.3	4
Groundcherry	9	—	—	—	1.0	40	—	—	—	—	—	720	.11	.04	2.8	11
Guava, common	23	289	4	13	.9	42	155	105	30	—	—	280	.05	.05	1.2	242
Guava, strawberry	23	289	4	—	.9	42	155	105	30	—	—	90	.03	.03	.6	37
Haw, scarlet	—	—	—	—	—	—	—	—	—	—	—	—	—	—	—	—
Jackfruit	22	407	2	—	—	38	—	—	—	—	—	40	.03	—	.4	8
Jujube, fresh	29	269	3	—	.7	37	—	—	—	—	—	—	.02	.04	.9	69
Jujube, dried	79	531	—	—	1.8	100	—	—	—	—	—	—	—	—	—	13
Kumquat	63	236	7	—	.4	23	18	125	—	—	—	600	.08	.10	—	36
Lemon, peeled	26	138	2	—	.6	16	—	—	31	—	—	20	.04	.02	.1	53
Lemon, with peel	61	145	3	—	.7	15	—	—	—	—	—	30	.05	.04	.2	77
Lemon, juice	7	141	1	8	.2	10	—	—	—	.005	—	20	.03	.01	.1	46

Fruit	Calcium Mgs	Potassium Mgs	Sodium Mgs	Magnesium Mgs	Iron Mgs	Phosphorus Mgs	Chlorine Mgs	Sulfur Mgs	Silicon Mgs	Iodine Mgs	Bromine Mgs	Vitamin A I.U.	Thiamine (B-1) Mgs	Riboflavin (B-2) Mgs	Niacin Mgs	Ascorbic Acid (C) Mgs
Lime	33	102	2	—	.6	18	265	224	—	—	—	10	.03	.02	.2	37
Lime juice	9	104	1	—	.2	11	—	—	—	—	—	10	.02	.01	.1	32
Loganberry	35	170	1	25	1.2	17	—	—	—	.016	—	200	.03	.04	.4	24
Longan, fresh	10	—	—	—	1.2	42	—	—	—	—	—	—	—	—	—	6
Longan, dried	45	—	—	—	5.4	196	—	—	—	—	—	—	.04	—	—	28
Loquat	20	348	—	—	.4	36	—	—	—	—	—	670	—	—	—	1
Lychee, fresh	8	170	3	—	.4	42	—	—	—	—	—	—	—	.05	—	42
Lychee, dried	33	1100	3	—	1.7	181	—	—	—	—	—	—	—	—	—	—
Mamey	11	47	15	—	.7	11	—	—	—	—	—	230	.02	.04	.4	14
Mango	10	189	7	18	.4	13	155	147	—	—	—	4800	.05	.05	1.1	35
Muskmelons:																
Cantaloupe	14	251	12	16	.4	16	—	—	—	—	9.45	3400	.04	.03	.6	33
Casaba	14	251	12	—	.4	16	—	—	—	—	9.45	30	.04	.03	.6	13
Honeydew	14	251	12	—	.4	16	—	—	—	—	9.45	40	.04	.03	.6	23
Nectarine	4	294	6	13	.5	24	—	—	—	—	—	1650	—	—	—	13
Olive, pickled:																
Green	61	55	2400	22	1.6	17	—	—	—	—	—	300	—	—	—	—
Ripe, Ascolano	84	34	813	—	1.6	16	—	—	—	—	—	60	trace	trace	—	—
Ripe, Mission	106	27	750	—	1.7	17	—	—	—	—	—	70	trace	trace	—	—
Ripe, Sevillano	74	44	828	—	1.6	20	—	—	—	—	—	60	trace	trace	—	—
Olive oil	0	0	0	0	0	0	0	0	25	0	0	—	—	—	—	0
Orange, peeled	41	200	1	11	.4	20	29	200	—	—	.46	200	.10	.04	.4	50
Orange with peel	70	196	2	—	.8	22	—	—	—	—	—	250	.10	.05	.5	71
Orange, peel only	161	212	3	—	.8	21	—	—	—	.002	.45	420	.12	.09	.9	136
Orange, juice	11	200	1	11	.2	17	—	—	—	—	—	200	.09	.03	.4	50
Papaw	—	—	—	—	—	—	—	—	—	—	—	—	—	—	—	—
Papaya	20	234	3	—	.3	16	—	—	—	—	—	1750	.04	.04	.3	56

Fruit	Calcium Mgs	Potassium Mgs	Sodium Mgs	Magnesium Mgs	Iron Mgs	Phosphorus Mgs	Chlorine Mgs	Sulfur Mgs	Silicon Mgs	Iodine Mgs	Bromine Mgs	Vitamin A I.U.	Thiamine (B-1) Mgs	Riboflavin (B-2) Mgs	Niacin Mgs	Ascorbic Acid (C) Mgs
Peach, fresh	9	202	1	10	.5	19	80	350	—	.016	.33	1330	.02	.05	1.0	7
Peach, dried	48	950	16	48	6.0	117	—	—	—	.009	—	3900	.01	.19	5.3	18
Pear, fresh	8	130	2	7	.3	11	—	145	38	—	.30	20	.02	.04	.1	4
Pear, dried	35	573	7	31	1.3	48	—	—	—	.006	—	70	.01	.18	.6	7
Persimmon, kaki	6	174	6	8	.3	26	—	—	—	—	—	2710	.03	.02	.1	11
Persimmon, native	27	310	1	—	2.5	26	270	415	—	—	—	—	—	—	—	66
Pineapple	17	146	1	13	.5	8	—	—	—	.002	—	70	.09	.03	.2	17
Pitanga (surinam cherry)	9	—	—	—	.2	11	—	—	—	—	—	1500	.03	.04	.3	30
Plantain	7	385	5	—	.7	30	—	—	—	—	—	—	.06	.04	.6	14
Plum, Damson	18	299	2	9	.5	17	—	103	68	.004	—	300	.08	.03	.5	—
Plum, Japanese	12	170	1	9	.5	18	—	103	68	.004	—	250	.03	.03	.5	6
Plum, prune type	12	170	1	9	.5	18	—	103	68	.004	—	300	.03	.03	.5	4
Pomegranate pulp	3	259	3	—	.3	8	34	20	—	—	—	trace	.03	.03	.3	4
Pricklypear	20	166	2	—	.3	28	—	—	—	—	—	60	.01	.03	.4	22
Prune, dried	51	694	8	40	3.9	79	10	80	90	.003	—	1600	.09	.17	1.6	3
Prune, dehydrated	90	940	11	—	4.4	107	—	—	—	—	—	2170	.12	.22	2.1	4
Quince	11	197	4	—	.7	17	—	—	—	—	trace	40	.02	.03	.2	15
Raisin	62	763	27	35	3.5	101	210	255	—	.003	—	20	.11	.08	.5	1
Raspberry, black	30	199	1	30	.9	22	—	—	—	—	.45	trace	.03	.09	.9	18
Raspberry, red	22	168	1	20	.9	22	290	1150	—	—	.45	130	.03	.09	.9	25
Roseapple	29	—	—	—	1.2	16	—	—	—	—	—	130	.02	.03	.8	22
Sapodilla	21	193	12	—	.8	12	—	—	—	—	—	60	trace	.02	.2	14
Sapote	39	—	—	—	1.0	28	—	—	—	—	—	410	.01	.02	1.8	20
Soursop	14	265	14	—	.6	27	—	—	—	—	—	10	.07	.05	.9	20
Strawberry	21	164	1	12	1.0	21	110	205	783	.019	.71	60	.03	.07	.6	59

	Cal-cium Mgs	Potas-sium Mgs	Sod-ium Mgs	Magne-sium Mgs	Iron Mgs	Phos-phorus Mgs	Chlo-rine Mgs	Sul-fur Mgs	Sili-con Mgs	Iodine Mgs	Bro-mine Mgs	Vita-min A I.U.	Thia-mine (B-1) Mgs	Ribo-flavin (B-2) Mgs	Nia-cin Mgs	Ascor Acid (C) Mgs
Fruit																
Sugarapple (sweetsop)	22	275	11	—	.6	41	—	—	—	—	—	10	.10	.14	1.0	34
Tamarind	74	781	51	—	2.8	113	—	—	—	—	—	30	.34	.14	1.2	2
Tangelo juice	—	—	—	—	—	—	—	—	—	—	.53	—	—	—	—	27
Tangerine	40	126	2	—	.4	18	—	—	—	—	—	420	.06	.02	.1	31
Tangerine, juice	18	178	1	—	.2	14	—	—	—	—	—	420	.06	.02	.1	31
Towelgourd	19	—	—	—	.9	33	—	—	—	—	—	380	.03	.04	.4	8
Watermelon	7	100	1	8	.5	10	110	210	160	.040	26.20	590	.03	.03	.2	7
Waxgourd	19	111	6	—	.4	19	—	—	—	—	—	0	.04	.11	.4	13
Seed																
Pumpkin & Squash	51	—	—	—	11.2	1144	—	—	—	—	—	70	.24	.19	2.4	—
Safflower	—	—	—	—	—	0	—	—	—	—	—	—	—	—	—	—
Safflower, oil	0	0	0	0	0	0	—	—	—	—	—	—	0	0	0	0
Sesame, whole	1160	725	60	181	10.5	616	—	—	—	—	—	30	.98	.24	5.4	0
Sesame, hulled	110	0	0	—	2.4	592	—	—	—	—	—	—	.18	.13	5.4	0
Sesame, oil	0	0	0	0	0	0	—	—	—	—	—	—	0	0	0	0
Sunflower	120	920	30	38	7.1	837	90	87	554	—	—	50	1.96	.23	5.4	—
Sunflower oil	0	0	0	0	0	0	—	—	—	—	—	—	0	0	0	0

Nut	Calcium Mgs	Potassium Mgs	Sodium Mgs	Magnesium Mgs	Iron Mgs	Phosphorus Mgs	Chlorine Mgs	Sulfur Mgs	Silicon Mgs	Iodine Mgs	Bromine Mgs	Vitamin A I.U.	Thiamine (B-1) Mgs	Riboflavin (B-2) Mgs	Niacin Mgs	Ascorbic Acid (C) Mgs
Almond	234	773	4	270	4.7	504	6	96	4	.002	—	0	.24	.92	3.5	trace
Beechnut	—	—	—	—	—	—	103	103	113	—	—	—	—	—	—	—
Brazilnut	186	715	1	225	3.4	693	85	433	—	—	—	trace	.96	.12	1.6	—
Butternut	—	—	—	—	6.8	—	—	—	—	—	—	—	—	—	—	—
Cashew	38	464	15	267	3.8	373	—	—	—	—	—	100	.43	.25	1.8	—
Chestnut, fresh	27	454	6	41	1.7	88	—	300	4	.002	—	—	.22	.22	.6	1
Chestnut, dried	52	875	12	—	3.3	162	1	—	—	—	—	—	.32	.38	1.2	3
Coconut cream	15	324	4	—	1.8	126	—	—	—	.009	—	0	.02	.01	.5	0
Coconut meat	13	256	23	46	1.7	95	320	85	—	—	—	0	.05	.02	.5	2
Coconut meat, dry	26	588	—	90	3.3	187	—	—	—	—	—	0	.06	.04	.6	2
Coconut milk	16	—	—	—	1.6	100	—	—	—	—	—	0	.03	trace	.8	—
Coconut water	20	147	25	28	.3	13	—	—	—	—	—	—	trace	trace	.1	—
Filbert	209	704	2	184	3.4	337	60	446	—	.002	—	—	.46	—	.9	trace
Hickory	trace	—	—	160	2.4	360	—	—	—	—	—	0	.34	.11	—	—
Macadamia	48	264	—	—	2.0	161	—	—	—	—	—	130	.86	.13	1.3	0
Pecan	73	603	trace	142	2.4	289	—	—	—	—	—	—	.62	—	.9	2
Pignolia	—	—	—	—	—	—	—	—	—	—	—	—	—	—	—	—
Pilinut	140	489	3	—	3.4	554	—	—	—	—	—	40	.88	.09	.5	trace
Pinon	12	—	—	—	5.2	604	—	—	—	—	—	30	1.28	23	4.5	trace
Pistachio	131	972	—	158	7.3	500	—	—	—	—	—	230	.67	—	1.4	0
Walnut, black	trace	460	3	190	6.0	570	—	—	—	—	—	300	.22	.11	.7	—
Walnut, English	99	450	2	131	3.1	380	12	22	12	.003	—	30	.33	.13	.9	2
Waterchestnut, Chinese	4	500	20	12	.6	65	15	45	—	—	—	0	.14	.20	1.0	4

Vegetable	Calcium Mgs	Potassium Mgs	Sodium Mgs	Magnesium Mgs	Iron Mgs	Phosphorus Mgs	Chlorine Mgs	Sulfur Mgs	Silicon Mgs	Iodine Mgs	Bromine Mgs	Vitamin A I.U.	Thiamine (B-1) Mgs	Riboflavin (B-2) Mgs	Niacin Mgs	Ascorbic Acid (C) Mgs
Artichoke, globe	51	430	43	—	1.3	88	206	260	530	.018	.98	160	.08	.05	1.0	12
Asparagus	22	278	2	20	1.0	62	510	536	950	.030	2.02	900	.18	.20	1.5	33
Bamboo shoots	13	533	—	—	.5	59	—	—	—	—	—	20	.15	.07	.6	4
Beet, common red	16	335	60	25	.7	33	295	50	200	.009	.34	20	.03	.05	.4	10
Beet, greens	119	570	130	106	3.3	40	—	—	—	—	—	6100	.10	.22	.4	30
Broccoli	103	382	15	24	1.1	78	275	3530	—	.003	—	2500	.10	.23	.9	113
Brussels sprouts	36	390	14	29	1.5	80	—	—	—	—	—	550	.10	.16	.9	102
Cabbage, Chinese	43	253	23	14	.6	40	—	—	—	.016	—	150	.05	.04	.6	25
Cabbage, common	49	233	20	13	.4	29	1045	1710	110	.009	1.05	130	.05	.05	.3	47
Cabbage, red	42	268	26	—	.8	35	1051	958	38	—	—	40	.09	.06	.4	61
Cabbage, savoy	67	269	22	—	.9	54	1003	1041	607	—	—	200	.05	.08	.3	55
Cabbage, spoon	165	306	26	—	.8	44	—	—	—	—	—	3100	.05	.10	.8	25
Carrot	37	341	47	23	.7	36	318	445	166	.012	1.40	11000	.06	.05	.6	8
Cauliflower	25	295	13	24	1.1	56	310	1186	337	—	.70	60	.11	.10	.7	78
Celeriac	43	300	100	—	.6	115	845	295	210	—	.42	—	.05	.06	.7	8
Celery	39	341	126	22	.3	28	1780	650	430	.007	17.60	240	.03	.03	.3	9
Chard, Swiss	88	550	147	65	3.2	39	740	690	530	.099	—	6500	.06	.17	.5	32
Chayote	13	102	5	—	.5	26	—	—	—	—	—	20	.03	.03	.4	19
Chervil	—	—	—	—	—	—	—	—	—	—	—	—	—	—	—	—
Chicory	18	182	7	13	.5	21	275	270	—	—	—	trace	.06	.10	—	22
Chicory greens	86	420	—	—	.9	40	—	—	—	—	—	4000	.08	.13	.5	56
Chive	69	250	—	32	1.7	44	232	666	—	—	—	5800	.16	.31	1.7	152
Collards, leaves	250	450	—	57	1.5	82	—	—	—	.017	—	9300	.20	.31	1.7	92
Collards, leaves and stems	203	401	43	48	1.0	63	112	368	50	.005	.31	6500	.15	.12	1.7	12
Corn, sweet	3	280	trace	—	.7	111	—	—	—	—	—	400	0	0	0	0
Corn, oil	0	0	0	0	0	0	—	—	—	—	—	—	—	—	—	0

Vegetable	Calcium Mgs	Potassium Mgs	Sodium Mgs	Magnesium Mgs	Iron Mgs	Phosphorus Mgs	Chlorine Mgs	Sulfur Mgs	Silicon Mgs	Iodine Mgs	Bromine Mgs	Vitamin A I.U.	Thiamine (B-1) Mgs	Riboflavin (B-2) Mgs	Niacin Mgs	Ascorbic Acid (C) Mgs
Cress	81	606	14	—	1.3	76	—	—	—	—	—	9300	.08	.26	1.0	69
Cucumber w/skin	25	160	6	11	1.1	27	660	690	800	.037	4.00	250	.03	.04	.2	11
Dandelion greens	187	397	76	36	3.1	66	347	288	917	—	—	14000	.19	.26	—	35
Dock (sorrel)	66	338	5	—	1.6	41	870	1330	—	.017	—	12900	.09	.22	.5	119
Eggplant	12	214	2	16	.7	26	670	445	—	—	—	10	.05	.05	.6	5
Endive (escarole)	81	294	14	10	1.7	54	—	—	—	—	—	3300	.07	.14	.5	10
Fennel	100	397	—	—	2.7	51	—	—	—	—	—	3500	—	—	—	31
Garlic	29	529	19	36	1.5	202	—	—	—	—	.44	trace	.25	.08	.5	15
Horseradish, raw	140	564	8	34	1.4	64	818	1984	818	—	—	—	.07	—	—	81
Horseradish, prepared	61	290	96	—	.9	32	—	—	—	—	—	—	—	—	—	—
Jerusalem artichoke	14	—	—	11	3.4	78	210	270	—	—	.62	20	.20	.06	1.3	4
Kale, leaves	249	378	75	37	2.7	93	1050	8600	—	—	—	10000	.16	.26	2.1	186
Kale, leaf & stem	179	378	75	—	2.2	73	—	—	—	.026	—	8900	—	—	—	125
Kohlrabi	41	372	8	37	.5	51	410	735	205	—	—	20	.06	.04	.3	66
Leek	52	347	5	23	1.1	50	310	740	740	—	.30	40	.11	.06	.5	17
Lettuce:																
Boston, Bibb	35	264	9	—	2.0	26	570	580	2400	.013	1.90	970	.06	.06	.3	8
Cos, Looseleaf	68	264	9	—	1.4	25	740	690	530	—	—	1900	.05	.08	.4	18
Iceberg, N.Y.	20	175	9	11	.5	22	1382	687	1464	—	—	330	.06	.06	.3	6
Mushroom	6	414	15	13	.8	116	57	250	65	.043	1.90	trace	.10	.46	4.2	3
Mustard greens	183	377	32	27	3.0	50	—	—	—	—	—	7000	.11	.22	.8	97
Mustard spinach	210	—	—	—	1.5	28	—	—	—	—	—	9900	—	—	—	130
N.Z. spinach	58	795	159	40	2.6	46	—	—	—	—	—	4300	.04	.17	.6	30
Okra	92	249	3	41	.6	51	—	710	—	.022	—	520	.17	.21	1.0	31

Vegetable	Cal-cium Mgs	Potas-sium Mgs	Sod-ium Mgs	Magne-sium Mgs	Iron Mgs	Phos-phorus Mgs	Chlo-rine Mgs	Sul-fur Mgs	Sili-con Mgs	Iodine Mgs	Bro-mine Mgs	Vita-min A I.U.	Thia-mine (B-2) Mgs	Ribo-flavin (B-2) Mgs	Nia-cin Mgs	Ascor Acid (C) Mgs
Onion, green	51	231	5	—	1.0	39	—	—	—	—	—	2000	.05	.05	.4	32
Onion, mature dry	27	157	10	12	.5	36	135	265	810	.014	.16	40	.03	.04	.2	10
Onion, Welsh	18	—	—	—	—	49	—	—	—	—	—	—	.05	.09	.4	27
Parsley	203	727	45	41	6.2	63	—	—	—	—	—	8500	.12	.26	1.2	172
Parsnip	50	541	12	32	.7	77	1040	800	960	—	1.30	30	.08	.09	.2	16
Pepper:																
Hot green	10	—	—	—	.7	25	—	—	—	—	—	770	.09	1.06	1.7	235
Hot red raw	29	1201	373	—	1.2	78	—	—	—	—	—	21600	.22	.36	4.4	369
Hot red dry	130	213	13	18	7.8	240	—	—	—	.019	—	77000	.23	1.33	10.5	12
Sweet green	9	—	—	—	.7	22	—	—	—	—	—	420	.08	.08	.5	128
Sweet red	13	—	—	—	.6	30	—	—	—	—	—	4450	.08	.08	.5	204
Potato w/skin	7	407	3	34	.6	53	155	289	88	.012	.63	trace	.10	.04	1.5	20
Pumpkin	21	340	1	12	.8	44	30	173	527	—	—	1600	.05	.11	.6	9
Purslane leaves	103	—	—	—	3.5	39	—	—	—	—	—	2500	.03	.10	.5	25
Radish, common	30	322	18	15	1.0	31	1000	715	100	—	.83	10	.03	.03	.3	26
Radish, oriental	35	180	—	—	.6	26	—	—	—	—	—	10	.03	.02	.4	32
Rhubarb	96	251	2	16	.8	18	681	234	346	—	.82	100	.03	.07	.3	9
Rutabaga	66	239	5	15	.4	39	100	530	—	.020	—	580	.07	.07	1.1	43
Salsify	47	380	—	—	1.5	66	160	560	—	—	—	10	.04	.04	.3	11
Seaweed, agar	567	—	—	—	6.3	22	—	—	—	.166	—	—	—	—	—	—
Seaweed, dulse	296	8060	2085	220	150.0	267	—	—	—	8.000	—	—	—	—	—	—
Seaweed, irishmos	885	2844	2892	—	8.9	157	—	—	—	—	—	—	—	—	5.7	—
Seaweed, kelp	1093	5273	3007	760	100.0	240	1221	930	—	150.0	—	2	—	.33	—	—
Seaweed, laver	—	—	—	—	—	—	—	—	—	—	—	trace	—	—	—	—
Shallot	37	334	12	—	1.2	60	—	—	—	—	.52	trace	.06	.02	.2	8
Spinach	93	470	71	88	3.1	51	1130	1245	810	.036	—	8100	.10	.20	.6	51

Vegetable	Cal-cium Mgs	Potas-sium Mgs	Sod-ium Mgs	Magne-sium Mgs	Iron Mgs	Phos-phorus Mgs	Chlo-rine Mgs	Sul-fur Mgs	Sili-con Mgs	Iodine Mgs	Bro-mine Mgs	Vita-min A I.U.	Thia-mine (B-1) Mgs	Ribo-flavin (B-2) Mgs	Nia-cin Mgs	Ascor Acid (C) Mgs
Squash:																
Summer (yellow, scallop and zucchini)	28	202	1	16	.4	29	—	—	—	.062	—	410	.05	.09	1.0	22
Winter (acorn, butternut and hubbard)	22	369	1	17	.6	38	—	—	—	—	—	3700	.05	.11	.6	13
Swamp cabbage	73	150	—	—	2.5	51	—	—	—	—	—	6300	.07	.12	.7	32
Sweet potato	32	243	10	31	.7	47	550	105	140	.010	—	8800	.10	.06	.6	21
Taro:																
Corms & tubers	28	514	7	—	1.0	61	—	—	—	—	—	20	.13	.04	1.1	4
Leaves & stems	76	—	—	—	1.0	—	—	—	—	—	—	—	—	—	—	31
Tomato, green	13	244	3	14	.5	27	1800	500	175	.010	2.00	270	.06	.04	.5	20
Tomato, red ripe	13	244	3	20	.5	27	830	1210	140	.025	1.20	900	.06	.04	.7	23
Turnip	39	268	49	58	.5	30	—	438	—	.076	4.25	trace	.04	.07	.6	36
Turnip greens	246	—	—	—	1.8	58	—	—	—	—	—	7600	.21	.39	.8	139
Vinespinach (basella)	109	—	—	—	1.2	52	—	—	—	—	—	8000	.05	—	.5	102
Watercress	151	282	52	20	1.7	54	775	5390	—	—	—	4900	.08	.16	.9	79
Yam, tuber	20	600	—	—	.6	69	—	—	—	—	—	trace	.10	.04	.5	9
Yambean, tuber	15	—	—	—	.6	18	—	—	—	—	—	trace	.04	.03	.3	20

Legume	Calcium Mgs	Potassium Mgs	Sodium Mgs	Magnesium Mgs	Iron Mgs	Phosphorus Mgs	Chlorine Mgs	Sulfur Mgs	Silicon Mgs	Iodine Mgs	Bromine Mgs	Vitamin A I.U.	Thiamin (B-1) Mgs	Riboflavin (B-2) Mgs	Niacin Mgs	Ascorbic Acid (C) Mgs
Bean:																
Lima, fresh	52	650	2	67	2.8	142	50	310	—	.005	—	290	.24	.12	1.4	29
Lima, dried	72	1529	4	180	7.8	385	4	260	—	.005	—	trace	.48	.17	1.9	—
Mung, dried	118	1028	6	—	7.7	340	—	—	—	—	—	80	.38	.21	2.6	—
Mung, sprouts	19	223	5	—	1.3	64	—	—	—	—	—	20	.13	.13	.8	19
Pinto, dried	135	984	10	163	6.4	457	—	—	—	—	—	—	.84	.21	2.2	—
Red, dried	110	984	10	—	6.9	406	—	—	—	.014	—	20	.51	.20	2.3	—
Snap, green	56	243	7	32	.8	44	710	1275	—	—	—	600	.08	.11	.5	19
Snap, yellow	56	243	7	32	.8	43	—	—	—	—	—	250	.08	.11	.5	20
White, dried	144	1196	19	170	7.8	425	69	130	25	—	—	0	.65	.22	2.4	—
Broadbean, fresh	27	471	4	—	2.2	157	—	—	—	—	—	220	.28	.17	1.6	30
Broadbean, dried	102	—	—	—	7.1	391	—	—	—	—	—	70	.50	.30	2.5	—
Chickpea, dried (garbanzo)	150	797	26	—	6.9	331	95	110	—	—	—	50	.31	.15	2.0	—
Cowpea, fresh	27	541	2	55	2.3	172	—	—	—	—	—	370	.43	.13	1.6	29
Cowpea, dried	74	1024	35	230	5.8	426	60	360	—	—	—	30	1.05	.21	2.2	—
Lentil, dried	79	790	30	80	6.8	377	150	120	—	—	1.00	40	.37	.22	2.0	—
Peanut, w/skin	69	674	5	206	2.1	401	23	45	—	.020	—	—	1.14	.13	17.2	0
Peanut, no skin	59	674	5	206	2.1	409	—	—	5	—	—	0	.99	.13	15.8	0
Peanut, oil	0	0	0	0	0	0	—	—	—	—	—	—	0	0	0	0
Pea, edible podded	62	170	—	—	.7	90	—	—	—	—	—	680	.28	.12	—	21
Pea, green fresh	26	316	2	35	1.9	116	140	600	—	—	—	640	.35	.14	2.9	27
Pea, dry	64	1005	35	180	5.1	340	53	103	127	.001	.21	120	.74	.29	3.0	—
Pigeonpea, fresh	42	552	5	—	1.6	127	—	—	—	—	—	140	.40	.17	2.2	39
Pigeonpea, dried	107	981	26	121	8.0	316	—	—	—	—	—	80	.32	.16	3.0	—

SOURCE: *Composition of Foods*, Agricultural Research Service, United States Dept. of Agriculture, Washington, D.C. 1975: U.S. Govt. Printing Office.

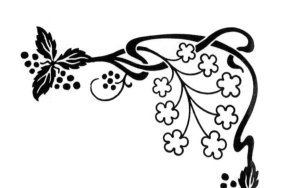

Appendix C:
Summary of Vitamins

Appendix C—Summary of Vitamins

Vitamin	Principal Synonyms	Main Biological Functions	Deficiency Symptoms	Main Sources	Average Daily Requirement
Vitamin A	Antixerophthalmic factor; Antiinfective factor Vitamin A$_1$ Vitamin A$_2$	Maintenance of healthy epithelial cells, formation of visual purple in retina	Xerophthalmia— night blindness, epithelial keratinization, failure of growth	Fish liver oil, butter, eggs, green and yellow vegetables	5,000 I.U. 1.2 mg. Vit. A acetate
Thiamine	Vitamin B$_1$ Antineuritic factor Antiberiberi factor	Metabolism of carbohydrates	Beriberi, polyneuritis	Yeast, whole cereal grains, lean pork	1–2 mg.
Riboflavin	Vitamin B$_2$ Vitamin G Anticheilosis factor	Oxidation in the tissues	Impaired growth, sore lips, cheilosis, vision defects	Yeast, liver	2–3 mg.

Nicotinic acid	Niacin P-P factor Antipellagra factor Antiblacktongue factor	Carbohydrate, fat, and protein metabolism	Pellagra, blacktongue disease in dogs	Yeast, wheat germ, liver	10–30 mg.
Pyridoxine	Vitamin B_6 Antidermatitis factor	Metabolism of amino acids	Dermatitis in rats	Yeast, rice polishings, eggs,	1.5 mg.
Pantothenic acid	Chick antidermatitis factor	Transfer of acyl radical, metabolism	Dermatitis and gray hair in animals	Yeast, liver, peanuts, eggs	2 mg.
Biotin	Vitamin H Anti-egg white injury factor	Carboxylation and decarboxylation reactions	Alopecia in rats	Peanuts, liver, kidney, eggs	0.2–0.6 mg.
Inositol	Mouse antialopecia factor Rat antispectacled eye factor	Normal growth of mice, rats, and chicks	Alopecia in mice	Muscle, liver, kidney, brain	
Choline	Growth factor	Lipotropic function, synthesis of acetylcholine	Fatty liver in animals	Egg yolk, soybeans, brain, liver, kidney	

Vitamin	Other names	Function	Deficiency	Sources	Daily requirement
Para-aminobenzoic acid	Anti-gray hair factor	Maintenance of normal fur coat	Gray hair in rats and mice	Yeast, liver	
Folic acid	Pteroylglutamic acid; antianemia factor	Red blood cell formation	Macrocytic anemic, growth retardation	Liver, kidney, dried beans, nuts, yeast	0.5–1.0 mg.
Vitamin B_{12}	Cyanocobalamin	Red cell formation, nucleic acid synthesis	Pernicious anemia	Liver, yeast	mg. quantities
Vitamin C	Ascorbic acid Antiscorbutic vitamin; Cevitamic acid	Maintenance of normal intercellular tissue, oxidation-reduction reactions	Scurvy, hemorrhages of skin and gums, teeth defects	Citrus fruit, raw leafy vegetables, tomatoes, peppers	70–80 mg.
Vitamin D	Antirachitic vitamin; Vitamin D_2 or calciferol (irradiated ergosterol) Vitamin D_3 (irradiated 7-dehydrocholesterol)	Calcium and phosphorus metabolism, bone and tooth formation	Rickets, defective tooth structure	Fish liver oil, egg yolks, irradiated ergosterol, action of sunlight	400–800 I.U. 10–20 g. calciferol

Vitamin E	α, β, and Tocopherol Antisterility factor Fertility vitamin	Normal muscle metabolism and fertility in animals	Sterility, muscular dystrophy in animals	Wheat germ oil, corn and cottonseed oils, green leafy vegetables, egg yolk, meat	6 mg.
Vitamin K	Vitamin K_1 Antihemorrhagic vitamin Coagulation vitamin	Production of prothrombin	Hemorrhage, increased clotting time for blood	Alfalfa, kale, spinach, cabbage	1–10 mg.

Table 15. SOURCE: *The Merck Manual of Diagnosis and Therapy, 1972.*

Bibliography

Childbirth

Benson, Ralph C. *Handbook of Obstetrics and Gynecology*. Los Altos, Calif.: Lange Medical Publications, 1974.

Dick-Read, Grantly. *Childbirth Without Fear*. New York: Harper & Row, 1953.

Eiger, Marvin, and Sally Olds. *The Complete Book of Breastfeeding*. New York: Bantam Books, 1972.

Elolesser, Leo, Edith Galt, and Isabel Hemingway. *Pregnancy, Childbirth and the Newborn: A Manual for Rural Midwives*. Ninos Heroes, Mexico: Inter-American Indian Institute, 1973.

Khan, Hazrat Inayat. *The Sufi Message of Hazrat Inayat Khan*. Vol. III. London: Barrie & Jenkins, 1971.

La Leche League. *The Womanly Art of Breastfeeding*. Franklin Park, Ill.: La Leche League, 1963.

May, Ina. *Spiritual Midwifery*. Summertown, Tenn.: Book Publishing Company, 1975.

Myles, Margaret. *Textbook for Midwives*. New York: Longmans, 1974.

Ostrander, Sheila, and Lynn Schroeder. *Natural Birth Control*. New York: Bantam Books, 1973.

Sousa, Marion, *Childbirth at Home*. New York: Bantam Books, 1976.

Food and Nutrition

Altman, Nathaniel, *Eating for Life*. Wheaton, Ill.: Theosophical Publishing House, 1973.

Beiler, Henry G., M.D. *Food Is Your Best Medicine*. London: Neville Spearman, 1968.

Borsook, Henry, Ph.D., M.D. *Vitamins: What They Are and How They Can Benefit You*. New York: Pyramid Books, 1971.

Clark, Linda. *Get Well Naturally.* New York: Arco, 1965.

Colimore, Benjamin and Sarah. *Nutrition and Your Body.* La Canada, Calif.: New Age Press, 1974.

Heritage, Ford, B.S.M.E. *Composition and Facts about Foods and Their Relationship to the Human Body.* Mokelumne Hill, Calif.: Health Research, 1971.

Davis, Adelle. *Let's Get Well.* Bergenfield, N.J.: New American Library, 1965.

Deal, Sheldon C., N.D., D.C. *New Life through Nutrition.* Tucson, Ariz.: New Life Publishing, 1974.

Heindel, Max. *New Age Vegetarian Cookbook.* Oceanside, Calif.: Rosicrucian Fellowship, 1968.

Hurd, Frank and Rosalie. *A Good Cook—Ten Talents.* Chisholm, Minn., Dr. and Mrs. Frank Hurd, 1968.

Kushi, Michio. *The Book of Macrobiotics.* Elmsford, N.Y.: Japan Publications Trading Company (USA), 1976.

Lee Foundation for Nutritional Research. *Portfolio of Reprints for the Doctor.* Milwaukee, Wisc.: Lee Foundation for Nutritional Research, 1974.

Lust, John. *Raw Juice Therapy.* Wellingborough, Northants, England: Thorson's Publishers, 1974.

New Age Vegetarian Cookbook, 4th ed. Oceanside, Calif.: The Rosicrucian Fellowship, 1973.

Newman, Laura. *Make Your Juicer Your Drug Store.* New York: Benedict Lust Publications, 1972.

Niethammer, Carolyn. *American Indian Food and Lore.* London: Collier Macmillan Publishers, 1974.

Nutrition Search, Inc. *Nutrition Almanac.* Hightstown, N.J.: McGraw Hill, 1975.

Ohsawa, Lima. *The Art of Just Cooking.* Kanagawa, Calif.: Autumn Press, 1974.

Passwater, Richard. *Supernutrition.* New York: Simon & Schuster, 1975.

Robertson, Laurel, Carol Flinders, and Bronwen Godfrey. *Laurel's Kitchen: A Handbook for Vegetarian Cookery and Nutrition.* Berkeley, Calif.: Nilgiri Press, 1977.

Rodale, Robert, ed. *The Encyclopedia of Organic Gardening.* Emmaus, Pa.: Rodale Books, 1971.

Rosenberg, Harold and A. N. Feldzamen. *The Doctor's Book of Vitamin Therapy.* Bronx, N.Y.: Vita Chart, 1976.

Shurtleff, William and Akiko Aoyagi, *The Book of Miso.* Kanagawa, Calif.: Autumn Press, 1976.

Stebbing, Lionel, ed. *Honey as Healer.* Sussex, England: Emerson Press, 1975.

Synder, Arthur W., Ph.D. *Foods That Preserve the Alkaline Reserve.* Los Angeles: Hansen's, n.d.

Walker, N.W. *Raw Vegetable Juices.* New York: Pyramid Books, 1970.

Warmbrand, Max. *The Encyclopedia of Health and Nutrition*. New York: Pyramid Publications, 1962.

Weiner, Michael A. *Earth Medicine—Earth Foods*. New York: Macmillan, 1972.

Herbology

Bach, Edward, M.B., B.S., D.P.H. *Heal Thyself: An Explanation of the Real Cause and Cure of Disease*. London: C. W. Daniel, 1974.

———. *The Twelve Healers and Other Remedies*. London: C. W. Daniel, 1975.

Bianchini, Francesco and Francesco Corbetta. *Health Plants of the World: Atlas of Medicinal Plants*. New York: Newsweek Books, 1977.

Chancellor, Philip, ed. *Handbook of the Bach Flower Remedies*. London: C. W. Caniel, 1971.

Christopher, John. *The Incurables*. New York: Crown, 1976.

———. *School of Natural Healing*. Provo, Utah: Dr. John Christopher, 1976.

Culpeper, Nicholas. *Culpeper's Complete Herbal*. New York: Sterling, 1959.

Dunmire, John R., ed. *Sunset Western Garden Book*. Menlo Park, Calif.: Lane Magazine and Book Company, 1973.

Edinger, Philip, ed. *How to Grow Herbs:* A Sunset Book. Menlo Park, Calif.: Lane Books, 1974.

Gerard, John. *The Herbal or General History of Plants*. New York: Dover, Reprint of 1633 edition, 1975.

Gonzales, Dr. Pedro Alvarez. *Yerbas Medicinales: Como Curarse con Plantas*. University of Mexico, Mexico City, Mexico, n.d.

Grieve, Mrs. M. *A Modern Herbal*. Vols. I and II. New York: Dover, 1971.

Harper-Shove, Lt.-Col. F. *Prescriber and Clinical Repertory of Medicinal Herbs*. Bradford, England: Health Science Press, 1952.

Heffern, Richard. *The Complete Book of Ginseng*. Millbrae, Calif.: Celestial Arts, 1976.

Heffern, Richard. *The Herb Buyer's Guide*. New York: Pyramid, 1975.

Herb Society of America. *The Herbarist*. Boston: 1974.

"Herb Ratings by the FDA." *Health Foods Business*. June 1978.

Hutchens, Alma R. *Indian Herbalogy of North America*. Ontario, Canada: Merco, 1974.

Jackson, Mildred and Terri Teague. *The Handbook of Alternatives to Chemical Medicine*. Oakland, Calif.: Terri K. Teague and Mildred Jackson, 1975.

Kirk, Donald R. *Wild Edible Plants of the Western United States*. Healdsburg, Calif.: Naturegraph Publishers, 1975.

Kloss, Jethro. *Back to Eden*. New York: Lancer Books, 1971.

Lucas, Richard. *Secrets of the Chinese Herbalists*. Englewood Cliffs, N.J.: Prentice-Hall, 1977.

Lust, John. *The Herb Book.* New York: Bantam, 1974.

Meyer, Joseph. *The Herbalist.* New York: Sterling, 1960.

Meyer, Joseph E., and Clarence Meyer. *The Herbalist.* Meyerbooks, 1960.

Nature's Herb Company. *Herbs and Spices for Home Use.* San Francisco, Calif.: n.d.

Park Seed Flowers and Vegetables. Greenwood, N.C.: 1977.

Pelt, J. M., and Younos, J. C. "Plantes medicinales et drogues de L'Afghanistan." *Extract from Bulletin de la Sociètè de Pharmacie de Nancy, No. 66* (September 1965).

Powell, Eric F., Ph.D., N.D. *The Modern Botanic Prescriber.* London: L. N. Fowler, 1971.

————. *The Natural Home Physician.* Sussex, England: Health Science, 1975.

Rose, Jeanne. *Herbs & Things.* New York: Grosset & Dunlap, 1974.

Royal, Penny C. *Herbally Yours.* Provo, Utah: Bi-World Publishers, 1976.

Shook, Dr. Edward E., N.D., D. C. *Advanced Treatise on Herbology.* Moke-lumne Hill, Calif.: Health Research, 1974.

Sweet, Muriel. *Common Edible and Useful Plants of the West.* Healdsburg, Calif.: Naturegraph, 1962.

"Taxonomist and Toxicologist" (Pamphlet). J. A. Duke, Presented at Second Annual Meeting of Herb Trade Association, Santa Cruz, California, September 15, 1978.

Thomson, Robert. *Natural Medicine.* New York: McGraw Hill, 1978.

Thomson, Samuel. *Guide to Health, or Botanic Family Physician.* Boston: J. Q. Adams, 1835.

Thomson, William A. R. *Medicines from the Earth.* Maidenhead, England: McGraw-Hill (UK), 1978.

Wren, R. W., ed. *Potter's New Cyclopedia of Medicinal Herbs and Preparations.* New York: Harper & Row, 1972.

History and Philosophy of Natural Medicine

Boyd, Doug. *Rolling Thunder.* New York: Dell, 1974.

Brock, J. Arthur, trans. *Greek Medicine, Being Extracts Illustrative of Medical Writers from Hippocrates to Galen.* New York: Dutton, 1972.

Healing Canadian Whole Earth Almanac, Vol. 2, No. 3. (Fall). Toronto: Canadian Whole Earth Research Foundation, 1971.

Illich, Ivan. *Medical Nemesis.* Westminster, Md.: Random House, 1976.

Kulvinskas, Viktoras. *Survival Into the 21st Century.* Wethersfield, Conn.: Omangod Press, 1976.

Spicer, Edward H. *Ethnic Medicine in the Southwest.* Tucson: University of Arizona Press, 1977.

Weil, Andrew, M.D. *The Natural Mind.* Boston: Houghton Mifflin, 1972.

Homeopathy

Boericke, William. *Materia Medica with Repertory.* New Delhi, India: B. Jain, 1927.

Chapman, J. B. *Dr. Schuessler's Biochemistry: A Medical Book for the Home.* Northants, England: Thorson's., 1961.

Coulter, Harris. *Homoeopathic Medicine.* St. Louis, Mo.: Formur, 1972.

Cowperthwaite, A. C. *A Text-Book of Materia Medica and Therapeutics.* New Delhi, India: B. Jain, 1976.

Hahnemann, Samuel. *The Lesser Writings.* Boulder, Colo.: Hermes, 1977.

———. *The Organon of Medicine.* Boulder, Colo.: Hermes, 1977.

Kent, J. T. *Lectures on Homoeopathic Materia Medica.* Calcutta, India: Sett Dey, 1971.

———. *Lectures on Homoeopathic Philosophy,* Calcutta, India: Sett Dey, 1974.

———. *Repertory of the Homoeopathic Materia Medica.* New Delhi, India: B. Jain, 1974.

Iridology

"Instructor's Manual for Research & Development." Dr. Bernard Jensen, D.C., N.D., Escondido, Calif.: Iridologists International, Volume 1, Issues 1–5, 1978.

Jensen, Bernard, D.C., N.D. *Chart for Iridology.* Solana Beach, Calif.: Jensen's Nutritional & Health Products, n.d.

———. *The Joy of Living and How to Attain It.* Solana Beach, Calif.: Bernard Jensen Products, 1970.

———. *The Science and Practice of Iridology.* Escondido, Calif.: Bernard Jensen, 1974.

Lindlahr, Henry. *Iridiagnosis and Other Diagnostic Methods.* Mokelumne Hill, Calif.: Health Research, 1922.

Wilborn, Robert, and James and Marcia Terrell. *Handbook of Iridiagnosis and Rational Therapy.* Mokelumne Hill, Calif.: Health Research, 1961.

Islamic Healing

Al-Ghazzali. *The Mysteries of Fasting.* Lahore, Pakistan: Ashraf, 1968.

———. *The Mysteries of Purity.* Lahore, Pakistan: Ashraf, 1970.

———. *The Alchemy of Happiness.* Lahore, Pakistan: Ashraf, 1964.

Begg, W. D. *The Big Five of India in Sufism.* Ajmer, India: W. D. Begg, 1972.

———. *The Holy Biography of Hazrat Khwaja Muinuddin Chishti.* Tucson, Ariz.: Chishti Order of America, 1977.

Gohlman, William E. *The Life of Ibn Sina.* New York: State University of New York Press, 1974.

Gruner, O. Cameron, M.D. *A Treatise on The Canon of Medicine of Avicenna,* Incorporating a Translation of the First Book. New York: Augustus M. Kelley, 1970.

Khan, Hazrat Inayat. *The Book of Health.* London: Sufi Publishing, 1962.

_____. *The Sufi Message of Hazrat Inayat Khan.* Vol. IV. London: Barrie & Jenkins, 1961.

Nicholson, R. A., trans. *Kashf Al-Mahjub of Al-Hujwiri.* London: Luzac, 1970.

Magnetics

Bagnall, Oscar. *The Origin and Properties of the Human Aura.* New York: Weiser, 1970.

Crabb, Riley, ed. *Radionics.* Boulder Creek, Calif.: University of the Trees Press, 1976.

Kilner, Walter. *The Human Aura.* New York: University Books, 1965.

Lewis, Roger. *Color and the Edgar Cayce Readings.* Virginia Beach, Va.: ARE Press, 1973.

Reichenbach, Karl von. *The Odic Force: Letterson Od and Magnetism.* New York: Universe Books, 1968.

Russell, Edward. *Report on Radionics.* London: Neville Spearman, 1973.

Natural Healing Systems

Abrams, Albert. *New Concepts in Diagnosis and Treatment.* Mokelumne Hill, Calif.: Health Research, 1922.

Airola, Paavo O., N.D. *Health Secrets from Europe.* New York: Arco, 1970.

_____. *How to Get Well.* Phoenix, Ariz.: Health Plus, 1976.

Barlow, Wilfred. *The Alexander Technique.* Westmister, Md.: Random House, 1973.

Bates, W. H. *Better Eyesight Without Glasses.* New York: Pyramid, 1975.

Benjamin, Harry. *Better Sight without Glasses.* London: Health for All Publishing Company, 1929.

Biron, W. A., B. F. Wells, and R. H. Houser. *Chiropractic Principles and Technic.* Chicago: National College of Chiropractic, 1939.

Borderland Sciences. *The Lakhovsky Multi-Wave Oscillator.* Vista, Calif.: Borderland Sciences Research Foundation, n.d.

Bragg, Paul. *The Miracle of Fasting.* Santa Ana, Calif.: Health Science, n.d.

Bricklin, Mark. *Natural Healing.* Emmaus, Pa: Rodale Press, 1976.

Carter, Mildred. *Hand Reflexology: Key to Perfect Health.* Englewood Cliffs, N.J.: Prentice-Hall, 1975.

_____. *Helping Yourself with Foot Reflexology.* Englewood Cliffs, N.J.: Prentice-Hall, 1975.

Ehret, Arnold. *Mucusless Diet Healing System.* Beaumont, Calif.: Ehret, 1922.

Garten, M. O., D.C. *The Health Secrets of a Naturopathic Doctor.* New York: Lancer, 1967.

Ingham, Eunice. *Stories the Feet Can Tell.* Rochester, N.Y.: Ingham, 1938.

Jarvis, D.C. *Folk Medicine.* San Francisco, Calif.: Rams Head, 1974.

Lakhovsky, Georges. *The Secret of Life.* Mokelumne Hill, Calif.: Health Research, 1935.

Law, Donald. *A Guide to Alternative Medicine.* New York: Doubleday, 1976.

Lindlahr, Henry, M.D. *Philosophy of Natural Therapeutics,* Vol. 1, Chicago: Lindlahr Publishing, 1922.

Mermet, Abbe. *Principles and Practice of Radiesthesia.* London: Watkins, 1935.

Naprapathic Principles. Chicago: Chicago College of Naprapathy, 1942.

Perry, Edward L., M.D. *Luyties Homeopathic Practice.* St. Louis, Mo.: Formur, 1976.

Sherman, Ingrid, Ph.D., Pss.D., N.D., D. O. (GB). *Natural Remedies for Better Health.* Healdsburg, Calif.: Naturegraph, 1970.

Smith, Oakley. *Naprapathic Technique.* Chicago: Chicago College of Naprapathy, 1933.

Stoddard, Alan. *Manual of Osteopathic Practice.* London: Hutchinson, 1969.

_____. *Manual of Osteopathic Technique.* London: Hutchinson, 1962.

Thie, John and Mary Marks. *Touch for Health.* Marina Del Rey, Calif.: DeVorss, 1973.

Vogel, Virgil J. *American Indian Medicine.* New York: Ballantine, 1973.

Walther, David S., D.C. *Applied Kinesiology.* Pueblo, Colo.: Systems D.C., 1976.

Wendel, Paul. *Diseases of the Stomach and Intestines Naturopathic.* Brooklyn, N.Y.: Wendel, n.d.

_____. *Standardized Naturopathy.* Brooklyn, N.Y.: Wendel, 1951.

Wigmore, Ann. *Be Your Own Doctor.* New York: Hemisphere, n.d.

Reference Works

Chen, Philip S. *Chemistry: Inorganic, Organic, and Biological.* New York: Barnes & Noble, 1968.

Compact Edition of the Oxford English Dictionary, Vols. I and II. Oxford: Oxford University Press, 1971.

Dick, William B. *Dick's Encyclopedia of Practical Receipts and Processes.* Leicester and Harriet Handsfield Edition. New York: Funk & Wagnalls, 1870.

Frohse, Franz, Max Brodel, and Leon Schlossberg. *Atlas of Human Anatomy.* New York: Barnes & Noble, 1970.

Gray, Henry. *Gray's Anatomy.* New York: Crown, 1977.

Guide Medica. *Enciclopedia Medica Per La Famiglia.* Volume VI. Milano, Italy: Proprieta Letteraria E. Artistica Riservata, 1964.

The Iconographic Encyclopedia of the Arts and Sciences. Philadelphia, Pa.: Iconographic, 1885.

"Instructions to Laboratory Users." N.R. Laboratory, Chicago: Uro-Biochemical Research, 1976.

Popenoe, Cris. *Wellness.* Washington, D.C.: Yes!, 1977.

Steen, Edwin B., and Ashley Montagu. *Anatomy and Physiology.* Vols. I and II. New York: Barnes & Noble, 1959.

Yokochi, C. *Photographic Anatomy of the Human Body.* Baltimore, Md.: University Park Press, 1971.

Spiritual Healing

Bailey, Alice A. *Esoteric Healing.* Vol. IV. New York: Lucis, 1953.

Bragdon, Claude. *A Primer of Higher Space (The Fourth Dimension).* Tucson, Ariz.: Omen, 1972.

Cayce, Edgar. *Medicines for the New Age.* Virginia Beach, Va.: Heritage Store, 1974.

deLaurence, L. W., *The Great Book of Magical Art, Hindu Magic and Indian Occultism.* Chicago: deLaurence, 1915.

Edwards, Harry. *A Guide to the Understanding and Practice of Spiritual Healing.* Guildford, Surrey, England: Spiritual Healing Sanctuary, 1974.

Gibbings, Cecil. *Divine Healing.* The Hague: East-West, 1976.

"A Guide to Spiritual & Magnetic Healing & Psychic Surgery in the Philippines." George W. Meek, Ft. Myers, Fla. no publication data.

Hall, Manly P. *Healing: The Divine Art.* Los Angeles, Calif.: Philosophical Research Society, 1971.

Heindel, Max. *Occult Principles of Health and Healing.* Oceanside, Calif.: Rosicrucian Fellowship, 1938.

Heline, Corinne. *Healing and Regeneration through Music.* Oceanside, Calif.: New Age 1965.

———. *Healing and Regeneration through Color.* Oceanside, Calif.: New Age, 1967.

Holy Bible. Cambridge: Cambridge University Press, n.d.

Kubler-Ross, Elizabeth. *Death.* Englewood Cliffs, N.J.: Prentice-Hall, 1975.

The Medical Group. Theosophical Research Center, London. *The Mystery of Healing.* Wheaton, Ill.: Theosophical Publishing House, 1968.

Mensendieck, Bess. *Look Better, Feel Better.* New York: Harper & Row, 1954.

Moody, Raymond. *Life After Life.* New York: Bantam Books, 1975.

Osborn, T. L. *Healing the Sick.* Tulsa, Okla.: OSFO, 1959.

Paramandanda, Swami. *Spiritual Healing.* Cohasset, Mass.: Vedanta Centre, 1975.

Sherman, Harold. *"Wonder" Healers of the Philippines.* Marina Del Rey, Calif.: DeVorss, 1966.

Szekely, Edmund Bordeaux, trans. *The Essene Gospel of Peace.* San Diego, Calif.: Academy, 1975.

_____. *The Essene Science of Life: According to the Essene Gospel of Peace.* San Diego, Calif.: Academy, 1975.

Worrall, Olga. *Olga Worral.* New York: Harper & Row, 1975.

Traditional Internal Medicine

A Barefoot Doctor's Manual (American Translation of the Official Chinese Paramedical Manual). Philadelphia, Pa.: Running Press, 1977.

Browne, E. G. *Arabian Medicine.* Cambridge, Mass.: Cambridge University Press, 1962.

Burang, Theodore. *Tibetan Art of Healing.* London: Watkins, 1974.

Cheng Man-Ch'ing and Robert W. Smith. *Tai-Chi.* Rutland, Vt.: Charles E. Tuttle, 1966.

Clausen, Torben, ed. *Practical Acupuncture,* San Mateo, Calif.: Cadre, 1973.

Evans-Wentz, W. Y. *The Tibetan Book of the Dead.* Fair Lawn, N.J.: Oxford University Press, 1960.

Garde, R. K., M.D. *Ayurveda for Health and Long Life.* Bombay, India: D. B. Taraporevala Sons, 1975.

Irwin, Yukiko and James Wagenvoord, *Shiatzu.* Philadelphia, Pa.: Lippincott, 1976.

Iyengar, B. K. S. *Light on Yoga.* New York: Schocken, 1977.

Kauz, Herman. *Tai Chi Handbook.* Garden City, N.Y.: Doubleday, 1974.

Leslie, Charles. *Asian Medical Systems.* Berkeley: University of California Press, 1976.

Traditional Eastern Medicine

Liu Zhaoyuan. *Acupuncture Charts.* Hong Kong: China Cultural Corp., 1975.

Lysebeth, Andre von. *Yoga Self Taught.* New York: Harper & Row, 1968.

Moss, Louis, M.D. *Acupuncture and You.* New York: Dell, 1972.

Namikoshi, Tokujiro. *Shiatsu Therapy.* Elmsford, N.Y.: Japan Publications Trading (USA), 1974.

Quinn, Joseph R., Ph.D., ed. *Medicine and Public Health in the People's Republic of China,* Bethesda, Md.: Geographic Health Studies, NIH, U.S. Dept. of HEW, 1973.

Rechung, Rinpoche. *Tibetan Medicine.* Bergenfield, N.J.: New American Library, 1974.

Thakkur, Chandrashekhar. *Introduction to Ayurveda.* New York: ASI, 1974.

Tohei, Koichi. *Aikido in Daily Life.* Elmsford, N.Y.: Japan Publications Trading (USA), 1966.

Veith, Ilza. *The Yellow Emperor's Classic of Internal Medicine.* Berkeley: University of California Press, 1973.

Vishnudevananda, Swami. *Complete Illustrated Book of Yoga.* New York: Simon & Schuster, 1960.

Unorthodox Cancer Therapies

Borderland Sciences. *The Koch Remedy for Cancer.* Vista, Calif.: Borderland Sciences Research Foundation, 1971.

Brown, Arlin J. *March of Truth on Cancer,* 7th ed. Fort Belvoir, Va.: Arlin J. Brown Information Center, 1971.

Cancer Control Journal. Vol. 3, No. 1 & 2. Los Angeles, Calif.: 1975.

Gerson, Max, M.D. *A Cancer Therapy: Results of Fifty Cases.* Del Mar, Calif.: Totality Books, 1975.

Griffin, Edward G. *World without Cancer, Parts I and II.* Westlake Village, Calif.: American Media, 1974.

Hendren, Julie S., pub. *Newsreal Series.* Issue No. 4 (August 1977).

Issels, Josef. *Cancer: A Second Opinion.* Kent, England: Hodder & Stoughton, 1975.

Kelley, William Donald, D.D.S., M.S. *One Answer to Cancer: An Ecological Approach to the Successful Treatment of Malignancy.* Grapevine, Calif.: Kelley Research Foundation, 1969.

Kittler, Glenn. *Laetrile, Control for Cancer.* New York: Warner Paperback Library, 1963.

Krebs, Ernest, et al. *The Laetriles-Nitrilosides in Prevention and Control of Cancer.* San Ysidro, Calif.: McNaughton Foundation, n.d.

Richardson, John, M.D., and Patricia Griffin, R.N. *Laetrile Case Histories: The Richardson Cancer Clinic Experience.* Westlake Village, Calif.: American Media, 1977.

Western Medicine

Blumhagen, Rex V., M.D., and Jeanne Blumhagen, M.D. *Family Health Care: A Rural Health Care Delivery Scheme.* Wheaton, Ill.: Medical Assistance Programs, 1974.

DeGowin, Richard L., and Elmer L. DeGowin. *Bedside Diagnostic Examination.* New York: Macmillan, 1969.

Goetz, John T., ed. *Advanced First Aid and Emergency Care* (The American National Red Cross). New York: Doubleday, 1973.

Gould, George M., A.M., M.D., and Walter L. Pyle, A.M., M.D. *Anomalies and Curiosities of Medicine.* New York: Sydenham, 1937.

———. *Pocket Cyclopedia of Medicine and Surgery.* Philadelphia, Pa.: Blakiston, 1926.

Haggard, Howard W., M.D., *Mystery, Magic and Medicine.* New York: Doubleday, Doran, 1933.

History of Pharmacy. (Pamphlet) New York: Parke, Davis, n.d.

Holvey, David N., M.D. (ed.). *The Merck Manual of Diagnosis and Therapy,* 12th ed. Rahway, N.J.: Merck, Sharp, & Dohme Research Laboratories, 1972.

Huff, Barbara, ed. *Physician's Desk Reference.* 30th ed. Oradell, N.J.: Medical Economics, 1976.

Wilson, John L. *Handbook of Surgery.* 4th ed. Los Altos, Calif.: Lange Medical Publications, 1969.

Windholz, Martha, ed. *The Merck Index: An Encyclopedia of Chemicals and Drugs.* 9th ed. Rahway, N.J.: Merck, 1976.

Wright, Harold N., M.S., Ph.D., and Mildred Montag, R.N., M.A. *A Textbook of Materia Medica Pharmacology and Therapeutics.* Philadelphia, Pa.: W. B. Saunders, 1945.

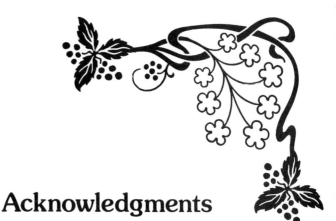

Acknowledgments

The author gratefully acknowledges permission to use the following material:

p. 4 (Acupuncture): Illustration from *Der goldene Schatz der chinesischen Medizin,* by Dr. Heinrich Wallnöfer and Anna von Rattauscher. Published by Schuler Verlagsgesellschaft, Stuttgart, 1959.

p. 13 (Astrology): Material from *Medical Astrology: How the Stars Influence Your Health,* by Omar V. Garrison. Published by Warner Paperback Library, New York, 1973. Permission granted by University Books, Inc.

pp. 14-15 (Avicenna): Material from *Natural Medicine,* by Dr. Robert Thomson. Published by McGraw-Hill, New York, 1978. Copyright © 1978 by Robert Thomson.

pp. 15-17 (Ayurveda): Material from *Ayurveda for Health and Long Life.* Published by D. B. Taraporevala Sons & Co. Private Ltd.

p. 16 (Ayurveda): Drawing by Amidhar Bhatt of Aurobindo Ashram, South India. Copyright © 1978 by Trewin Copplestone Publishing Ltd.

pp. 20-21 (Bach Flower Remedies): Excerpted from *The Bach Flower Remedies* (three books in one volume by Edward Bach, M.D., and F. J. Wheeler, M.D.). Copyright © by The Edward Bach Healing Center, and Keats Publishing, Inc.

p. 36 (C Vitamin): Material from *New Life Through Nutrition,* by Sheldon Deal, D.C., N.D. Published by New Life Publishing, 1974.

p. 56 (Cupping): Material from *Natural Medicine,* by Dr. Robert Thomson. Published by McGraw-Hill, New York, 1978. Copyright © 1978 by Robert Thomson.

pp. 97-101 (Herbalism): Material from *Herbology,* by F. Fletcher Hyde. Permission granted by F. Fletcher Hyde, President Emeritus, The National Institute of Medical Herbalists, U.K.

Acknowledgments   *282*

p. 102 (Hippocrates): Photograph courtesy of the Mansell collection, London.

pp. 103-104 (Homeopathy): Material from *Luyties Homeopathic Practice,* by Edward L. Perry. Published by Formur, Inc., 1974.

p. 104 (Homeopathy): Drawing courtesy Mary Evans, Picture Library.

pp. 116-20 (Iridology): Diagram of iris and eye chart from *Science and Practice of Iridology,* by Bernard Jensen, D.C.

pp. 150-51 (Miracle Cures): Material from "Miracles" selection in *The Holy Biography of Hazrat Khwaja Muinuddin Chishti,* by W. D. Begg. Published by Chishti Sufi Mission, 1979.

p. 189 (Rolfing): Illustration © 1958 by Ida Rolf.

Index